ABC of
Obesity

ABC of
Obesity

EDITED BY

Naveed Sattar
Professor of metabolic medicine, University of Glasgow

Mike Lean
Professor of nutrition, University of Glasgow

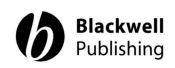
Blackwell Publishing

BMJ|Books

Blackwell Publishing, Inc., 350 Main Street, Malden, Massachusetts 02148-5020, USA
Blackwell Publishing Ltd, 9600 Garsington Road, Oxford OX4 2DQ, UK
Blackwell Publishing Asia Pty Ltd, 550 Swanston Street, Carlton, Victoria 3053, Australia

First published 2007

3   2008

Library of Congress Cataloging-in-Publication Data
ABC of obesity / edited by Naveed Sattar and Mike Lean.
    p. ; cm.
 "BMJ Books."
 Includes bibliographical references and index.
 ISBN 978-1-4051-3674-7 (alk. paper)
 1. Obesity--Great Britain. 2. Obesity--Prevention--Great Britain. I. Sattar, Naveed. II.
Lean, Mike.
 [DNLM: 1. Obesity--prevention & control--Great Britain. 2. Disease Outbreaks-
-prevention & control--Great Britain. 3. Health Policy--Great Britain. 4. Obesity--
complications--Great Britain. 5. Obesity--therapy--Great Britain. WD 210 A134 2007]
 RC628.A2356 2007
 362.196'39800941--dc22

                                                                    2006102879

ISBN 978-1-4051-3674-7

A catalogue record for this title is available from the British Library

Set by BMJ Electronic Production
Printed and bound in Singapore by Markono Print Media Pte Ltd

Commissioning Editor: Eleanor Lines
Editorial Assistant: Vicky Pittman
Development Editor: Sally Carter
Production Controller: Rachel Edwards
Senior Technical Editor: Julia Thompson
For further information on Blackwell Publishing, visit our website:
www.blackwellpublishing.com

Contents

Contributors

Sir George Alberti
Senior research fellow at Imperial College and emeritus professor of medicine, University of Newcastle Medical School

Alison Avenell
Chief Scientist Office career scientist, Health Services Research Unit, School of Medicine, University of Aberdeen

Christopher D Byrne
Professor of endocrinology and metabolism, University of Southampton

Nick Finer
Director of the Wellcome Clinical Research Facility, Addenbrooke's Hospital, Cambridge

Ian Greer
Professor of obstetrics and gynaecology, University of Glasgow

Laurence Gruer
Director of public health science, NHS Health Scotland

Thang S Han
Specialist registrar, department of diabetes and endocrinology, University College London Hospitals

David Haslam
General practitioner and clinical director, National Obesity Forum

James O Hill
Director of the Center for Human Nutrition, University of Colorado, USA

John G Kral
Professor of surgery and medicine, department of surgery, SUNY Downstate Medical Center, New York

Debbie A Lawlor
Professor of epidemiology, department of social medicine, University of Bristol

Jose Lara
Clinical research fellow, Division of Developmental Medicine, Human Nutrition, University of Glasgow

Mike Lean
Professor of nutrition, University of Glasgow

Colin S McArdle
Honorary professor, university department of surgery, Royal Infirmary, Glasgow

Donald C McMillan
Senior lecturer, university department of surgery, Royal Infirmary, Glasgow

Jane E Ramsay
Consultant obstetrician and gynaecologist, Ayrshire Maternity Unit, Kilmarnock

John J Reilly
Professor of paediatric energy metabolism, University Division of Developmental Medicine, Yorkhill Hospitals, Glasgow

Naveed Sattar
Professor of metabolic medicine, University of Glasgow

Sarah H Wild
Senior lecturer in epidemiology and public health, University of Edinburgh

David Wilson
Senior lecturer, Division of Child Life and Health, University of Edinburgh, Royal Hospital for Sick Children, Edinburgh

Foreword

Some 30 years ago a report from the Royal College of Physicians, London, predicted the consequences of inaction with regard to the emerging problems of overweight and obesity. The report and the almost loan voices of Garrow and James, the leading British researchers and clinicians of the day, went largely unheeded and the prophetic predictions have been fulfilled. Worse news, still, is the fact that the measures being undertaken have done little, if anything, to stem the tide of the epidemic of obesity and associated health consequences, especially type 2 diabetes, which is now prevalent in children as well as adults. The cost to individuals and to society is enormous and cannot be sustained; 3000 deaths per year in the United Kingdom, 18 million work days lost through illness, and an estimated annual cost attributable to obesity of £3.5 billion. From a global perspective the escalating rates of obesity and comorbidities in developing countries that are still struggling to cope with the consequences of undernutrition and infectious diseases are even more worrying than the situation in affluent countries. The obesity epidemic needs to be managed using principles similar to those invoked to deal with epidemics and pandemics of infectious diseases: intensive education programmes aimed at health professionals and the public, public health measures to halt or at least radically reduce the number of new cases, appropriate measures for the management of existing cases, an active research programme and overall central coordination. This series of papers edited and largely written by two of today's leading British researchers with other invited experts provides all the essential information for health professionals at all levels. The essays are clearly written and should also be compulsory reading for healthcare planners, those responsible for national policy, and politicians because regulatory and legislative measures will almost certainly be required to supplement existing measures aimed at stemming the tide of the obesity epidemic.

The World Health Organization Global Strategy on Diet, Physical Activity and Health sets the scene at an international level. However, little will be achieved without coordinated national action. This ABC series of essays tells readers "why" and provides clear direction as to "how". It is highly recommended.

Jim Mann
Professor in Human Nutrition and Medicine, Director of the Edgar
National Centre for Diabetes Research and WHO Collaborating
Centre for Human Nutrition, University of Otago, New Zealand

1 Obesity—time to wake up

David Haslam, Naveed Sattar, Mike Lean

The obesity epidemic in the United Kingdom is out of control, and none of the measures being undertaken show signs of halting the problem, let alone reversing the trend. The United States is about 10 years ahead in terms of its obesity problem, and it has an epidemic of type 2 diabetes with obesity levels that are rocketing. Obesity is a global problem—levels are rising all over the world. Moreover, certain ethnic groups seem to be more sensitive than others to the adverse metabolic effects of obesity. For example, high levels of diabetes and related diseases are found in South Asian and Arab populations. Although most of the medical complications and costs of obesity are found in adults, obesity levels are also rising in children in the UK and elsewhere.

Definition of obesity

- Obesity is excess body fat accumulation with multiple organ-specific pathological consequences
- Obesity is categorised by body mass index (BMI), which is calculated by weight (in kilograms) divided by height (in metres) squared. A BMI > 30 indicates obesity and it is reflected by an increased waist circumference
- Waist circumference is a better assessor of metabolic risk than BMI because it is more directly proportional to total body fat and the amount of metabolically active visceral fat

---

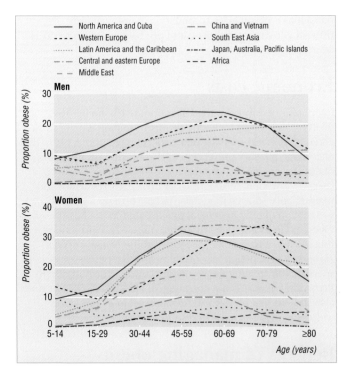

Prevalence of obesity worldwide. Adapted from Haslam D, James WP. *Lancet* 2005;366:1197-209

Limited time to act

Obesity can be dealt with using three expensive options:
- Treat an almost exponential rise in secondary clinical consequences of obesity
- Treat the underlying obesity in a soaring number of people to prevent secondary clinical complications
- Reverse the societal and commercial changes of the past 200 years, which have conspired with our genes to make overweight or obesity more normal.

Sheaves of evidence based guidelines give advice on the treatment of all the medical consequences of obesity, and an evidence base for identifying and treating obesity is accumulating. Although the principles of achieving energy balance are known, an evidence base of effective measures for preventing obesity does not exist. The methods of randomised clinical trials are inappropriate, and so some form of continuous improvement methodology is needed.

In the United Kingdom, even if preventive measures against obesity were successful immediately (so that not one more person became obese) and people who are obese do not gain weight, there would still be an epidemic of diabetes and its complications within 10-20 years. This is because so many young people are already in the clinically "latent" phase of obesity, before the clinical complications present. Treatment of obesity must be prioritised alongside prevention. It will take an unprecedented degree of cooperation between government departments; schools; food, retail, and advertising industries; architects and town planners; and other groups to improve our "toxic" environment. Meanwhile, in their clinics, doctors have to deal with the obesity epidemic one person at a time—a daunting role.

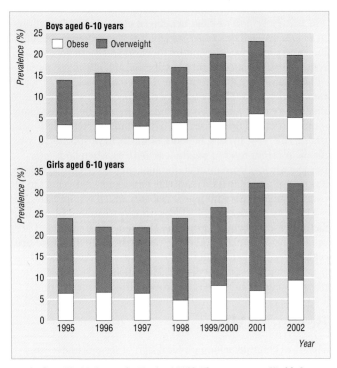

Results from Health Survey for England 2002. The most recent Health Survey for England (2004) states that "Between 1995 and 2001, mean BMI increased among boys (from 17.6 to 18.1) and girls (from 18.0 to 18.4) aged 2-15"

Health consequences

It has been known for centuries that obesity is the cause of serious chronic disease. Only relatively recently has the full spectrum of disease linked to obesity become apparent—for example, recognition that most hypertension, previously considered "essential," is secondary to obesity. Among preventable causes of disease and premature death, obesity is overtaking smoking.

Economic costs

Every year obesity costs the UK economy £3.5bn (€5.1bn, $6.4bn), and results in 30 000 deaths;18 million days of work taken off for sickness each year. Strategies for primary care that encourage primary prevention of chronic disease, including obesity management, would achieve considerable financial rewards. The Counterweight study on obesity reduction and maintenance showed that obese people take up a greater proportion of time in general practice than non-obese people. Obese patients also need more referral, and are prescribed more drugs across all the categories of the *British National Formulary* than people of normal weight. Resources are being spent mainly treating the secondary consequences of obesity. Preventing obesity is not encouraged. The Counterweight study also showed that obesity can be managed in a population without a major increase in resources.

Benefits of managing obesity

Uniquely among chronic diseases, obesity does not need a scientific breakthrough to be treated successfully. Enough is known about the causes of obesity and that diet, exercise, behaviour therapy, drugs, and even laparoscopic surgery can be effective. The barriers to successful management of obesity are political and organisational ones, along with a lack of resources. In the long term, the cheapest and most effective strategy to improve the health of the population may be to prioritise and provide incentives for the management of obesity.
The metabolic and vascular benefits of even modest reductions in weight are well described. Weight loss also enhances fertility in women, improves respiratory function and mental wellbeing, reduces risk of cancers and joint disease, and improves quality of life. Major benefits for individuals from dramatic interventions, like obesity surgery, have been shown. Optimal medical treatment can also produce major weight loss for many patients (outside the constraints of randomised controlled trials). The most striking benefits, however, in proportional terms, are from modest weight loss (5-10%), when fat is particularly lost from intra-abdominal sites. For example, this amount of weight loss increases life expectancy 3-4 years for overweight patients with type 2 diabetes, which is impressive.

Obesity management includes priority treatment of risk factors for cardiovascular disease. The benefits of treatment are greater for overweight and obese people because their risks are higher. Primary prevention of obesity and overweight would prevent much secondary disease. Many people do stay at normal weight, but there is no proven effective intervention.

Beyond BMI

The most clinically telling physical sign of serious underlying disease is increased waist circumference, which is linked to insulin resistance, hypertension, dyslipidaemia, a proinflammatory state, type 2 diabetes, and coronary heart

---

Health consequences of obesity

Greatly increased risk (relative risk >3)
- Diabetes
- Hypertension
- Dyslipidaemia
- Breathlessness
- Sleep apnoea
- Gall bladder disease

Moderately increased risk (relative risk about 2-3)
- Coronary heart disease or heart failure
- Osteoarthritis (knees)
- Hyperuricaemia and gout
- Complications of pregnancy—for example, pre-eclampsia

Increased risk (relative risk about 1-2)
- Cancer (many cancers in men and women)
- Impaired fertility/polycystic ovary syndrome
- Low back pain
- Increased risk during anaesthesia
- Fetal defects arising from maternal obesity

Costs attributable to obesity in Scotland in 2003*

Illness	GP contacts		Prescribing costs (£)	
	No	Cost (£)	Per person	Total
Obesity	58 346	758 503	3	2 818 025
Hypertension	988 493	12 850 406	179	43 650 190
Type 2 diabetes	65 777	855 098	409	18 901 220
Angina pectoris	93 178	1 211 309	720	20 348 921
Myocardial infarction	33 372	433 838	720	14 598 139
Osteoarthritis	37 003	481 045	112	2 240 485
Stroke	5829	75 777	35	106 333
Gallstones	1575	20 470	67	57 448
Colon cancer	2631	34 207	0	0
Ovarian cancer	382	4967	91	6970
Gout	17 321	225 170	25	244 155
Prostate cancer	0	0	2949	162 609
Endometrial cancer	0	0	168	14 362
Rectal cancer	0	0	1114	12 812
Total	1 303 907	16 950 791		103 161 670

£1 = €1.40 or US$1.8

* Adapted from Walker A. *The cost of doing nothing—the economics of obesity in Scotland*. University of Glasgow, 2003 (www.cybermedicalcollege.com/Assets/Acrobat/Obesitycosts.pdf)

Estimated metabolic and vascular benefits of 10% weight loss

Blood pressure
- Fall of about 10 mm Hg in systolic and diastolic blood pressure in hypertensive patients

Diabetes
- Fall of up to 50% in fasting glucose for newly diagnosed patients

People at risk for diabetes, such as those with impaired glucose tolerance
- >30% fall in fasting or two hour insulins
- >30% increase in insulin sensitivity
- 40-60% fall in incidence of diabetes

Lipids
- Fall of 10% in total cholesterol
- Fall of 15% in low density lipoprotein cholesterol
- Fall of 30% in triglycerides
- Rise of 8% in high density lipoprotein cholesterol

Mortality
- >20% fall in all cause mortality
- >30% fall in deaths related to diabetes
- >40% fall in deaths related to obesity

disease. More than 250 years ago, Giovanni Battista Morgagni used surgical dissection to show visceral fat. He linked its presence to hypertension, hyperuricaemia, and atherosclerosis. Jean Vague (in the 1940s and '50s) and Per Bjorntorp (in the 1980s) led the interest in gender specific body types of android and gynoid fat distribution. Pear shaped women tend to carry metabolically less active fat on their hips and thighs. Men generally have more central fat distribution, giving them an apple shape when they become obese, although obese women can have a similar shape.

Cross-sectional studies show that waist to hip ratio is a strong correlate of other diseases. Prospective studies, however, show a large waist as the strongest anthropometric predictor of vascular events and diabetes because it predicts risk independently of BMI, hip circumference, and other risk factors.

Management of obesity in the UK

Clinical practice in the UK focuses on secondary prevention for chronic diseases. Obesity is often neglected in evidence based approaches to managing its consequences. One problem is in recording the diagnosis.

Computerised medical records and better linking of datasets will help monitor efforts to reduce obesity locally and nationally. The UK Counterweight audit showed that height and weight are measured in about 70% of primary care patients only. The diagnosis of obesity is rarely recorded in reports from hospital admissions or outpatient attendance. A survey of secondary prevention of coronary heart disease shows that, despite the importance of obesity as a coronary heart disease risk factor, it is still poorly managed, even in high risk patients. Although patients with type 2 diabetes are often overweight, most are managed in primary care and few regularly see a dietician.

The first revision of the general medical services contract gives practices eight points for creating registers of obese adults, but this is only a start in readiness for a more emphatic second revision of the contract. BMI is seldom measured in people of normal weight so their progression to becoming overweight is missed, and with it the opportunity to prevent more than half of the burden of diabetes in the UK.

Producing a register of obese individuals is futile unless something is done with the list. Weight management and measurement of fasting lipid profile, glucose, and blood pressure should be encouraged. This could be used to identify people at high risk of cardiovascular disease and diabetes through risk factors related to obesity, which individually might fall below treatment thresholds. Without these steps the contract creates more work with no clinical benefit. The arguments are strong for awarding points for assessing obese individuals and offering weight management programmes. The clinical and economic benefit will be extended if effective obesity prevention strategies can be developed. These are not alternative strategies: strategies are needed for both prevention and treatment with ongoing monitoring and evaluation.

Conclusion

Obesity affects almost every aspect of life and medical practice. The rise in obesity and its complications threatens to bankrupt the healthcare system. Early treatment and prevention offer multiple long term health benefits, and they are the only way towards a sustainable health service. Doctors in all medical and surgical specialties can contribute.

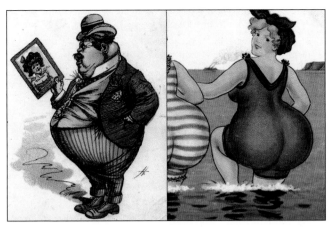

Stereotypical apple (metabolically harmful, more common in men) and pear (metabolically protective and more common in women) shapes. Making obesity an object of humour has impeded the understanding of its medical consequences. Obesity can contribute to musculoskeletal and psychological problems and have profound effects on quality of life

Further reading
- Haslam D, James WP. Obesity. *Lancet* 2005;366:1197-209.
- Torgerson JS, Hauptman J, Boldrin MN, Sjostrom L. XENical in the prevention of diabetes in obese subjects (XENDOS) study: a randomized study of orlistat as an adjunct to lifestyle changes for the prevention of type 2 diabetes in obese patients. *Diabetes Care* 2004;27:155-61.
- James WP, Astrup A, Finer N, Hilsted J, Kopelman P, Rossner S, et al. Effect of sibutramine on weight maintenance after weight loss: a randomized trial. STORM Study Group. Sibutramine Trial of Obesity Reduction and Maintenance. *Lancet* 2000;356:2119-25.
- McQuigg M, Brown J, Broom J, Laws RA, Reckless JP, Noble PA, et al. Counterweight Project Team. Empowering primary care to tackle the obesity epidemic: the Counterweight Programme. *Eur J Clin Nutr* 2005;59:93-100.
- De Bacquer D, De Backer G, Cokkinos D, Keil U, Montaye M, Ostor E, et al. Overweight and obesity in patients with established coronary heart disease: are we meeting the challenge? *Eur Heart J* 2004;25:121-8.
- Scottish Intercollegiate guidelines (www.sign.ac.uk)
- National Institute of Health guidelines (www.nhlbi.nih.gov/guidelines/obesity/ob_gdlns.htm)

The figure showing obesity in English girls and boys aged 6-10 uses data from Health Survey for England 2002 (using criteria of the International Obesity Task Force for overweight and obesity), and is adapted from British Medical Association Board of Science. *Preventing childhood obesity*, 2005 (www.bma.org). The box showing health consequences of obesity is adapted from International Obesity Taskforce (www.iotf.org/.../slides/IOTF-slides/sld016.htm). The box showing metabolic and vascular benefits of 10% weight loss is adapted from Jung RT. Obesity as a disease. *Br Med Bull* 1997;53:307-21.

Competing interests: DH has received honorariums for presentations and advisory board attendance from Sanofi-Aventis, Abbott, Roche and GlaxoSmithKline. NS has received fees for consulting and speaking from Sanofi-Aventis, GlaxoSmithKline, and Merck, and from several companies in the field of lipid lowering therapy. ML has received personal and departmental funding from most major pharmaceutical companies involved in obesity research, and from several food companies. A full list can be seen on www.food.gov.uk/science/ouradvisors/ACR/

2 Assessment of obesity and its clinical implications

Thang S Han, Naveed Sattar, Mike Lean

Obesity can be assessed in several ways. Each method has advantages and disadvantages, and the appropriateness and scientific acceptability of each method will depend on the situation.

The assessment methods often measure different aspects of obesity—for example, total or regional adiposity. They also produce different results when they are used to estimate morbidity and mortality. When there is increased body fat, there will also be necessary increases in some lean tissue, including the fibrous and vascular tissues in adipose tissue, heart muscle, bone mass, and truncal or postural musculature. All these non-fat tissues have a higher density (1.0 g/ml) than fat (0.7 g/ml). The density of non-fat tissues is also increased by physical activity, which of course tends to reduce body fat.

In general, measurements of body weight and body dimensions (anthropometry) are used to reflect body fat in large (epidemiological) studies or in clinic settings as such measurements provide a rapid and cheap way to estimate body fatness and fat distribution. Densitometry or imaging techniques are used in smaller scale studies such as clinical trials.

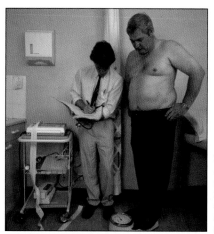

For weight measurement subjects should ideally be in light clothing and bare feet, fasting, and with empty bladder; repeat measures are best made at same time of day

Adolphe Quételet was a 19th century Belgian scientist who established the body mass index to classify people's ideal weight for their height

Anthropometry

Body mass index (BMI) has traditionally been used to identify individuals who are the most likely to be overweight or obese. It is calculated by dividing the weight (in kilograms) by the height (in metres) squared. Generally, a high value indicates excessive body fat and consistently relates to increased health risks and mortality. Unusually large muscle mass, as in trained athletes, can increase BMI to 30, but rarely above 32. BMI categories and cut-offs are commonly used to guide patient management. BMI reference ranges assume health in other aspects—healthy weight may be lower with major muscle wasting.

Waist circumference was developed initially as a simpler measure—and a potentially better indicator of health risk than BMI—to use in health promotion. Waist circumference is at least as good an indicator of total body fat as BMI or skinfold thicknesses, and is also the best anthropometric predictor of visceral fat.

Classification of body fatness based on body mass index according to World Health Organization

BMI	Classification
< 18.5	Underweight
18.5-24.9	Healthy
25-29.9	Overweight
30-39.9	Obese
≥ 40	Morbidly obese

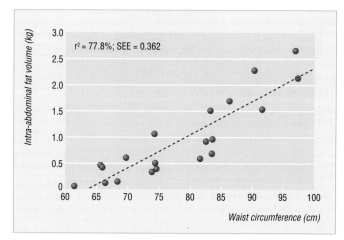

The correlation of visceral fat with waist circumference is strong. Adapted from Han TS et al. *Int J Obes Relat Metab Disord* 1997;21:587-93

Levels of health risks associated with waist circumference (cm), defined by waist circumference action levels in white men and women

Level	Men	Women	Health risk*
Below action level 1	< 94	< 80	Low
Action levels 1 to 2	≥ 94-101.9	≥ 80-87.9	Increased
Above action level 2	≥ 102	≥ 88	High

*Risk for type 2 diabetes, coronary heart disease, or hypertension.

People with increased fat around the abdomen or wasting of large muscle groups, or both, tend to have a large waist circumference relative to that of the hips (high waist to hip ratio). Waist circumference alone, however, gives a better prediction of visceral and total fat and of disease risks than waist to hip ratio. Waist circumference is minimally related to height, so correction for height (as in waist to height ratio) does not improve its relation with intra-abdominal fat or ill health.

BMI is still a useful guide to obesity related health risks, but waist circumference is a simple alternative with additional value for predicting metabolic and vascular complications

People with a large waist are many times more at risk of ill health, including features of metabolic syndrome (such as diabetes, hypertension, and dyslipidaemia) as well as shortness of breath and poor quality of life. These increased risks also apply in people whose BMI is normal but who have a large waist. However, BMI and waist circumference are colinear, so combining the two measures adds relatively little to risk predicton.

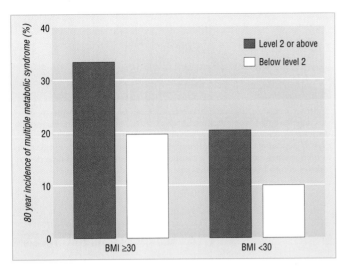

Incidence of metabolic syndrome in people with different categories of body mass index and of waist circumference action levels (action level 1=94 cm in men and 80 cm in women, action level 2=102 cm in men and 88 cm in women). Adapted from Han TS et al. *Obes Res* 2002;10:923-31

During weight loss, each kilogram of weight loss is equivalent to a reduction of 1 cm in waist circumference. However, there is greater measurement error for waist circumference, so body weight is the best measure for monitoring change.

Classification of overweight and obesity by body mass index, waist circumference, and associated disease risk* (adapted from data from National Institutes of Health)

	BMI	Risk relative to normal weight and waist circumference	
		Men <102 cm, women <88 cm	Men ≥102 cm, women ≥88 cm
Underweight	18.5	Not increased	Not increased
Normal	18.5-24.9	Not increased	Increased
Overweight	25.0-29.9	Increased	High
Obesity (class I)	30.0-34.9	High	Very high
Obesity (class II)	35.0-39.9	Very high	Extremely high
Extreme obesity (class III)	≥40.0	Extremely high	Extremely high

Most of the relevant information in relation to risk can be derived from measurement of waist alone.
*Disease risk for type 2 diabetes, hypertension, and cardiovascular disease.

Waist to hip ratio was introduced—mainly as a result of Swedish research—on the assumption that it would predict fat distribution better than waist circumference alone. Subsequent research, however, showed that it did not.

Hip circumference does have a relation to health and disease, but in an inverse way, such that a relatively large hip circumference is associated with lower risks of diabetes and coronary heart disease. This is probably because hip circumference reflects muscle mass, which is reduced in type 2 diabetes and inactivity.

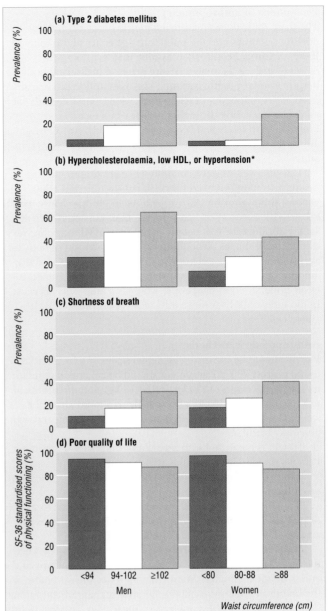

Prevalence of diabetes (a); hypercholesterolaemia, low HDL (high density lipoprotein), or hypertension (b); shortness of breath (c); and poor quality of life (d) in people with large waist. Adapted from Lean ME et al. *Lancet* 1998;351:853-6

Weight gain leads to greater adverse metabolic changes in certain ethnic groups. As a result, Asians should be considered overweight if BMI ≥23 and obese if BMI ≥27.5. Waist levels associated with risk are also lower in Asian men (≥90 cm v ≥94 cm in Europoids)

Waist to hip ratio and myocardial infarction

- A recent report from the international Interheart study proposed waist to hip ratio as the best adiposity risk marker for acute myocardial infarction
- The study was a case-control study, however, rather than prospective
- Lower hip circumference may have reflected lower muscle mass in cases, whereas the value of waist circumference may have been diminished in this study because a non-standard method was used
- These factors might have exaggerated the association between waist to hip ratio and myocardial infarction

Perceptions of anthropometry

The main difficulty with anthropometric measures is that doctors, scientists, and the public are not aware of the value of these measures. People often assume that technological devices—such as fat analysers—are better at measuring body fat, despite evidence to the contrary. This assumption often arises from better marketing of technology, yet no portable body fat analysers (including those that measure bioelectrical impedance, which is highly dependent of body hydration status) are better than waist circumference for measuring body fat in adults.

Cut-off levels of waist circumference relating to increased health risks have not been fully defined for different ethnic groups, although some African and Asian groups clearly have a greater risk of coronary heart disease than Europoids at the same cut-off levels. Two people of the same BMI may have very distinct body shapes, depending on the distribution of body fat and skeletal muscle. A change in single measures, such as the amount of weight loss or reduction in waist circumference, is easily understood by lay people, whereas a ratio (such as waist to hip ratio or BMI) is more difficult to conceptualise. BMI charts can help.

Anthropometric methods

Weight should be measured by digital scales or a beam balance to the nearest 100 g. Equipment should be calibrated regularly by standard weights (4×10 kg and 8×10 kg), and the results of test weighing recorded in a book. Patients should ideally be weighed in light clothing and bare feet, ideally fasting and with an empty bladder.

Height is measured with a regularly calibrated stadiometer. Patients stand in bare feet that are kept together. The head is level with a horizontal Frankfort plane (an imaginary line from lower border of the eye orbit to the auditory meatus).

If a patient cannot stand—for example, is confined to a chair or bed—BMI can still be derived from special equations using arm span or lower leg length instead of height.

Waist circumference should be measured midway between the lower rib margin and iliac crest, with a horizontal tape at the end of gentle expiration. Waist circumference measurement at the umbilical level is not reliable because sagging of abdominal skin occurs in very obese subjects or those who have lost weight previously.

Densitometry

Total body fat was classically measured by densitometry based on the Archimedes principles of water displacement, assuming just two body compartments: fat (density about 0.7 g/ml) and fat-free tissue (about 1.0 g/ml). Under this principle, if two individuals of the same weight on land have different proportions of body fat and lean tissue, the one with more body fat and less lean tissue would weigh less under water.

Imaging

In the past decade, new imaging techniques such as computed tomography and magnetic resonance imaging allow discrete deposits of body fat to be imaged. Specific fat depots can be measured, including the visceral fat depots. These relate more strongly than subcutaneous fat to metabolic abnormalities. Fat in other structures, such as the liver, or muscle cannot be quantified easily. Imaging is very expensive and can be problematic for people who are claustrophobic.

Precise and accurate measurements of regional fat mass can be estimated from two dimensional, transverse, multiple slices.

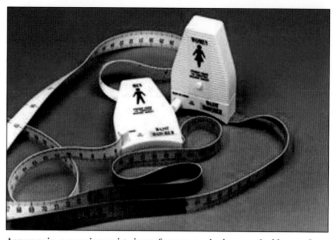

Accuracy in measuring waist circumference can be improved with use of a specially designed tape measure, although a change in body fat may not be detected by waist circumference in very fat people, when the abdominal fat mass is pendulous. During waist measurement, patients should be asked not to hold in their stomach, and a constant-tension, spring-loaded tape device reduces errors from over-enthusiastic tightening during measurement

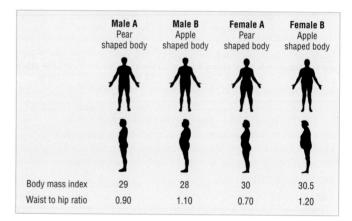

	Male A Pear shaped body	Male B Apple shaped body	Female A Pear shaped body	Female B Apple shaped body
Body mass index	29	28	30	30.5
Waist to hip ratio	0.90	1.10	0.70	1.20

Variation in human body fat distribution in men and women. In each pair of men and pair of women (subjects A and B), the body mass indices are similar. However, the waist circumference and waist to hip ratios of subjects B are much higher, indicating a greater distribution of body fat around the abdomen as well as a decreased amount of muscle mass around the hips

> **Densitometry requires underwater weighing facilities and takes time, so it is expensive; furthermore, many people would not like to be submerged in water. Densitometry is therefore not used routinely. It also cannot indicate body fat distribution**

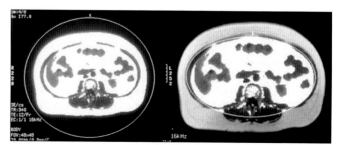

Images of different fat compartments by computed tomography. The inner elliptic ring shows intra-abdominal fat

The fat volume estimated from a single slice based on regression equations can be used to reduce time, cost, and risk of radiation exposure for some purposes, such as repeated studies in the same patient.

Other imaging techniques, including dual energy x ray examination, are good predictors of visceral fat but, like computed tomography, expose subjects to radiation which limits their use in repeated measurements. They were originally calibrated against densitometry.

Bioimpedance

Obese people have increased lean body mass as well as increased fat mass. Bioimpedance estimates total body water crudely, as a component of lean body mass. Therefore, estimation of fat mass by this technique is relatively weak.

Summary

Identifying people who are overweight, and particularly with accumulation of excessive visceral fat, is essential for directing future intervention. BMI and waist circumference are well validated and available to all health professionals. Waist circumference is arguably better, but both are simple, and change is best monitored by following body weight. "Black box" methods such as bioimpedance do not add greatly, and even more complex methods remain in the research domain.

The photo at the start of the article is published with permission from Simon Fraser/SPL. The computed tomograms were reproduced with permission from The American Diabetes Association (Kelly IE, Han TS, Walsh K, Lean ME. *Diabetes Care* 1999;22:288-93).

Comparison of relative strengths and weaknesses of body mass index versus waist circumference

BMI	Waist circumference
Predictor of total body fat and related health risks at a population level	Predictor of total body fat and related health risks at a population level
Weak relation to visceral fat	Best simple marker for visceral fat
Modest predictor of multiple health risks in individuals	Stronger predictor of multiple health risks in individuals
Routinely collected in general practitioner contracts	Not yet collected as part of general practitioner contracts
Large existing databases	Databases accumulating rapidly
Less reliable in discriminating health risk when BMI <30	Less reliable in discriminating health risks when BMI >40
Potentially confounded by differences in muscle mass	Larger measurement error than BMI
Requires shoes off	Requires upper clothing off
Sex differences ignored	Cut-offs different for men and women
Needs calculation or chart for clinical use; is conceptually complex	Easy home monitoring (no calculation needed); is easily understood

Key references and further reading

- Expert Panel on Detection, Evaluation, and Treatment of High Blood Cholesterol in Adults. Executive summary of the third report of the National Cholesterol Education Program (NCEP) Expert Panel on Detection, Evaluation, And Treatment of High Blood Cholesterol In Adults (Adult Treatment Panel III). *JAMA* 2001;285:2486-97.
- Han TS, Lean ME, Seidell JC. Waist circumference remains useful predictor of coronary heart disease. *BMJ* 1996;312:1227-8.
- Lean ME, Han TS, Morrison CE. Waist circumference as a measure for indicating need for weight management. *BMJ* 1995;311:158-61.
- Lissner L, Bjorkelund C, Heitmann BL, Seidell JC, Bengtsson C. Larger hip circumference independently predicts health and longevity in a Swedish female cohort. *Obes Res* 2001;9:644-6.
- Must A, Jaques PF, Dallal GE, Bajema CJ, Dietz WH. Long term morbidity and mortality of overweight adolescents: a follow-up of the Harvard growth study of 1922 to 1935. *N Engl J Med* 1992;327:1350-5.
- World Health Organization. *Global strategy on diet, physical activity and health.* www.who.int/dietphysicalactivity/publications/facts/ obesity/ (accessed 25 Jun 2006)
- National Heart, Lung, and Blood Institute. *The practical guide: identification, evaluation, and treatment of overweight and obesity in adults.* 2000. www.nhlbi.nih.gov/guidelines/obesity/practgde.htm (accessed 25 Jun 2006)
- WHO Expert Consultation. Appropriate body mass index for Asian populations and its implications for policy and intervention strategies. *Lancet* 2004;363:157-63.

3 Management: Part I—Behaviour change, diet, and activity

Alison Avenell, Naveed Sattar, Mike Lean

In the United Kingdom over 22% of the adult population is now obese, with multiple health problems related to a body mass index—weight (in kilograms) divided by height (in metres) squared—of 30 or higher. In England the national service frameworks for diabetes and coronary heart disease highlight the importance of helping patients who are obese. People continue to gain weight until their 50s and 60s, so 30-40% of older people will be obese, with chronic disease, mobility problems, and depression aggravated by obesity.

Obesity needs to be managed like any other chronic disease—with empathy and a non-judgmental professional attitude. Helping people to manage their weight is difficult and can be discouraging and time consuming for health professionals.

High relapse rates, apparent lack of effectiveness, and lack of training and resources are major obstacles. However, an increasing evidence base exists for the effective management of obesity. And resources for health professionals are also now available.

Resources for health professionals

- www.nationalobesityforum.org.uk (National Obesity Forum)
- www.domuk.org (Dietitians in Obesity Management UK)
- www.aso.org.uk (Association for the Study of Obesity)
- www.nice.org.uk/page.aspx?o = 296567 (draft guidance from National Institute for Health and Clinical Excellence) (accessed 1 Aug 2006)

For people who are obese, long term low fat diets—together with increased physical activity and strategies to help modify their lifestyle—may prevent type 2 diabetes in those with impaired glucose tolerance and improve the control of hypertension and type 2 diabetes. These health benefits are seen with surprisingly small weight losses—5-10% sustained over a year or more, well within achievable goals for weight loss and despite some weight regain over subsequent years.

General strategies for helping a patient with a weight problem include agreeing an individual, realistic, weight loss goal, such as 5-10% over three to six months. Achieving this goal can help motivate success. Aim for weight loss initially, followed by a distinct strategy for weight maintenance. Provide ongoing support and positive feedback; this can be provided in a group setting.

A careful history can provide useful information for weight management. Weight, height, body mass index, and waist circumference (plus cardiovascular risk factors if indicated) should be documented regularly—changes in strategy can be used to help to motivate the patient.

Aims and success criteria

The emphasis for "obesity treatment" used to be on weight loss. But, as identified in the 1996 Scottish Intercollegiate Guidelines Network guideline, weight loss is only one element in weight management. Management encompasses:

- Weight loss (short term, three to six months)
- Weight maintenance (long term, more than six months)
- Priority reduction of risk factors.

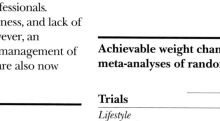

Achievable weight change (95% confidence intervals) from meta-analyses of randomised controlled trials in adults

Trials	Weight change (kg) at 1-3 years		
	1	2	3
Lifestyle interventions v control			
Deficit of 600 kcal/day,* or low fat diet	−5.3 (−5.9 to −4.8)	−2.4 (−3.6 to −1.2)	−3.6 (−4.5 to −2.6)
Diet and exercise	−4.8 (−5.4 to −4.2)	−2.7 (−3.6 to −1.8)	Not studied
Diet and behaviour therapy	−7.2 (−8.7 to −5.8)	−1.8 (−4.8 to 1.2)	Not studied
Diet, exercise, and behaviour therapy	−4.0 (−4.5 to −3.5)	−3.0 (−3.6 to −2.4)	−2.0 (−2.7 to −1.3)
Effect of adding exercise			
Adding exercise to diet	−2.0 (−3.2 to −0.7)	Not studied	−8.2 (−15.3 to −1.2)
Adding exercise to diet, plus behaviour therapy	−3.0 (−4.9 to −1.1)	−2.2 (−4.2 to −0.1)	Not studied
Effect of adding behaviour therapy			
Adding behaviour therapy to diet	−7.7 (−12.0 to −3.4)	Not studied	−2.9 (−8.6 to 2.8)

Data from Avenell et al (see Further Reading box).
*1 kcal = 4.18 kJ.

Important factors to evaluate in patient's history

- Is the weight problem recent or longstanding (for example, since childhood)?
- Consider the patient's successful and unsuccessful attempts at losing weight and establish what he or she thinks about them
- What is the patient's attitude to smoking? For example, he or she may not be interested in stopping smoking because they may feel they will gain weight
- How does the patient feel about illness and medication? For example, he or she may relate weight gain to inadequate thyroxine replacement, that weight gain is associated with depression
- Is there a family history of weight problems? Does the patient's partner have weight problems?
- Does the patient believe that their medical, social, or psychological problems are related to their obesity?
- What is the patient's motivation for weight loss or stability?

Successful weight management does not necessarily have to mean weight loss. It can also reflect weight maintenance in somebody who in the past has gained weight.

In general, the diet and lifestyle strategies to achieve weight loss, weight maintenance, and improved risk factors are the same. There may be individual variations in responses to individual components—for example, lower fat or lower carbohydrate diets, or for physical activity.

Behavioural change

The key elements to successful behavioural change are frequent contact and support. Group counselling does not seem less effective than individual counselling for long term weight change. Weight loss clubs may be helpful, but evidence is limited. For some people, however, initial individual counselling may be needed, and groups may not be beneficial—for example, for men needing support but whose local group comprises mainly women. If possible, immediate family or key friends should be involved. Beneficial behavioural changes may have knock-on effects for other members of the family.

Weight loss plans move through various stages: precontemplation, contemplation, preparation, action, maintenance, and often relapse. Patients need help to make plans with achievable goals—unrealistically high goals for weight loss lead to disappointment. The goals can be reviewed over time, with a graded approach to changing habits.

Commonly used techniques, such as self monitoring, identifying internal triggers for eating, and creation of coping strategies, can help with behaviour change. There is evidence that these techniques aid weight loss and maintenance. They have been incorporated into a successful model for weight management in primary care in the UK—the Counterweight programme. This programme achieved weight loss results similar to those achieved by the Diabetes Prevention Program Group (see Further Reading box) for those who completed the programme.

Prompts or reminders can be used to help to build better habits. A lapse presents an important opportunity to plan how to deal with the experience next time. Rewards should be planned, and evidence of benefit—in terms of reduction in cardiovascular risk factors or in changes in clothing size—can be helpful. It is important to help to build self esteem and avoid criticism. A diary of food intake and physical activity can prompt discussion about situations that led to a particular behaviour, so that strategies can be planned.

Web based resources are available for patients, and a Haynes manual (Banks I. *HGV man manual.* Yeovil: Haynes, 2005) has been produced specifically to help men to lose weight.

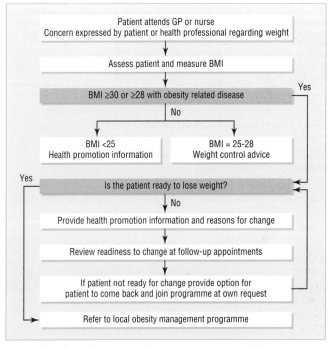

A possible pathway for starting weight management to provide support appropriate to the stage. Adapted from Counterweight programme (see Further Reading box)

Web based resources for patients to help with weight control

- www.realslimmers.com (online food retailer and diet club)
- www.eating4health.co.uk (organisation of state registered dietitians offering dietary advice and programmes)
- www.fatmanslim.com
- www.whi.org.uk (Walking the Way to Health Initiative—aims to get more people walking in their own communities)
- www.weightlossresources.co.uk (gives tips and programmes for losing weight)
- www.toast-uk.org (The Obesity Awareness and Solutions Trust—campaigning charity offering a help and information line via phone or email; online chat rooms and forum facilities)

Examples of commonly used behaviour modification techniques

Behavioural approach	Techniques
Self monitoring	Daily diary (time of eating, type and amount of food, thoughts and feelings, physical activity); personalised 5-10% weight loss targets; weight monitoring charts
Stimulus control	Patient to identify and record external and internal triggers for eating; negotiate goals (for example, if eats when worried or stressed, to make list of alternative, relaxing activities)
Eating behaviour	Negotiate goals (such as avoid watching television or reading while eating)
Cognitive restructuring	Realistic weight loss expectations of 5-10% discussed at first appointment; achievable dietary and activity goals set in collaboration with patient; patient encouraged to challenge self defeating thoughts with positive thoughts; patient discouraged from using words such as "always" and "never"
Nutrition education	Patient learns how to read food labels; patient learns about dietary goals
Relapse management	Patient encouraged to plan in advance how to prevent lapses; management of cravings discussed; patient encouraged to generate list of coping strategies for high risk situations

Diets

Dietitians with skills in weight management can give advice and support to general practices, including information for patients. Diets partly work by imposing a regular regimen. Regular meal times, and the need for breakfast, are important. People who skip meals early in the day often more than make up for this later in the day. Shift workers have particular problems, so it is important to help the patient make his or her own plan.

Snacking or grazing is best discouraged, but low energy snacks must be available when snacking is unavoidable. Reducing portion sizes, using portion controlled foods (including meal replacements) and limiting the size of plates used may all be helpful. Patients should be advised to avoid having tempting, high energy foods at home, to shop when they are not hungry, and to use a shopping list.

A diary of food intake is a useful starting point for making changes. This may be particularly useful for patients who claim to be unable to lose weight despite eating virtually nothing. A diary may help them to see that they eat more than they thought and is useful for looking at triggers to overeating.

New diets appear in the media and on the bookshelves all the time and it can be difficult to counter this barrage. Consistent evidence shows that a long term, low fat diet produces long term weight loss and beneficial changes in lipids, blood glucose, glycaemic control, and blood pressure. Typically, such a diet would have a deficit of 500-600 kcal/day below the current requirement for energy balance, leading to a weight reduction of 0.5 kg a week. A low fat diet can be consistent with providing low glycaemic index foods, as in diets that focus on eating foods with a low glycaemic index. Such a diet provides the best chance for a long term change to healthy eating habits, with protection against chronic diseases such as cancer and heart disease. Low energy meal replacements may be helpful for some patients, but palatability can be a problem.

Very low energy diets may produce better initial weight loss—which might improve motivation—but long term, the weight loss achieved in this way is rarely any greater than the loss achieved with low fat diets. Rapid weight loss may occasionally be required, however (for example, to allow surgery to proceed).

Low carbohydrate, Atkins-type diets (diets that focus on eating mostly protein, with small amounts of carbohydrate) are effective in the short term but less so after a few months. Short term side effects include headache, constipation, halitosis from ketosis, and fatigue. Longer term effects on disease risks have been little studied for these diets. Low carbohydrate diets lead to deterioration of some parts of the lipid profile—for example, low density lipoprotein cholesterol—but improvements in high density lipoprotein cholesterol, triglycerides, and glycaemic control. Short term use is unlikely to be harmful and can be a starting point for the otherwise poorly motivated patient.

Physical activity

Patients should be encouraged to reduce their inactivity rather than "do more exercise," which for some people may have negative connotations of team sports and "going to the gym." Weight loss and long term weight maintenance will be improved if activity levels can be increased. Step counters may be useful to set daily targets, but their value is unclear. As well as its effect on weight loss, increased physical activity has additional benefits for cardiovascular risk factors, insulin resistance, and depression and also limits the loss of lean tissue and contributes to bone health.

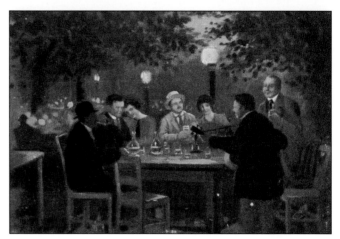

Some patients may find that alcohol accounts for a much larger energy intake than they expected. Alcohol can also encourage some people to eat more

Key principles for a successful diet

- Include a variety of foods from the main food groups
- Limit portion size
- Reduce the proportion of fat, particularly saturated fat
- Partially replace saturated fat with monounsaturated fat (such as olive oil) or omega 3 polyunsaturated fats
- Increase intake of fruit and vegetables to at least five portions a day
- Ensure that meals include wholegrain and high fibre foods, and foods with a low glycaemic index
- Reduce sugar intake
- Limit salt intake
- Follow a structured meal plan that starts with breakfast

Beans on toast, fruit, and porridge are all useful standbys for low energy meal replacements—and they are all easily available and tasty

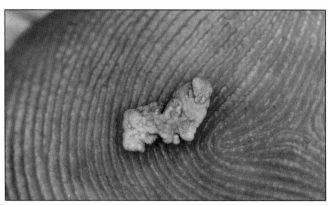

Concerns have been raised that diets focusing long term on eating mostly protein with small amounts of carbohydrate may increase the risk of osteoporosis and kidney stones (above)

Keeping physically active helps people to curb excess appetite and avoid situations that prompt eating

Patients who have previously been inactive must decide and plan for themselves how to incorporate more physical activity into their current lifestyle—for example, less sitting and more standing, less television, walking some of the way to work, gardening, and cycling. Walking initiatives in the patient's area may be useful (www.whi.org.uk). Patients may think that they have to go to exercise classes, but this may be unrealistic for their current activity levels and lifestyle. Other people may enjoy attending organised classes and the peer support this provides. Recording physical activity in a diary can be used in much the same way as a diet diary. Patients may find it difficult to attain the levels of moderate activity recommended initially, but this should be the long term goal. Although the Department of Health's recommended goals for physical activity clearly reduce the risk of cardiovascular disease for people who are overweight and obese, they are not sufficient to counteract all the ill effects of obesity.

Helping someone to change their behaviour to prevent or reduce obesity requires a flexible approach tailored to that individual, with encouragement when, inevitably, setbacks occur.

The authors thank Karen Allan for reviewing a previous draft of the article. The cycling photograph is published with permission from Dennis MacDonald/Alamy. The illustration of a drinking party is *Heurigen Party, Vienna* by Rudolf Klingsbogl, published with permission from *Vienna's Musical Sites* (1927). The photograph of the kidney stone is published with permission from Stephen J Kraemer/SPL.

Competing interests: In the past five years, Alison Avenell has received one fee for speaking from Roche Products UK, the manufacturer of orlistat.

Department of Health recommendations on physical activity for adults*

- Thirty minutes of at least moderate activity on at least five days a week
- For many people, 45-60 minutes of moderate activity a day may be necessary to prevent obesity
- People who have been obese and have managed to lose weight may need to do 60-90 minutes of activity daily to maintain weight loss
- Recommended levels of activity may be obtained in one session or as bouts of activity of 10 minutes or more
- The activity can be "lifestyle" activity (such as walking, cycling, climbing stairs, hoovering, mowing lawn), structured exercise, or sport

*www.dh.gov.uk/assetRoot/04/08/09/88/04080988.pdf (accessed 1 Aug 2006)

Further reading and resources

- Avenell A, Broom J, Brown TJ, Poobalan A, Aucott L, Stearns SC, et al. Systematic review of the long-term effects and economic consequences of treatments for obesity and implications for health improvement. *Health Technol Assess* 2004;8(21).
- Costain L, Croker H. Helping individuals to help themselves. *Proc Nutr Soc* 2005;64:89-96.
- Diabetes Prevention Program Group. Reduction in the incidence of type 2 diabetes with lifestyle intervention or metformin. *N Engl J Med* 2002;346:393-403.
- National Obesity Forum. *Managing obesity in primary care* [CD-Rom]. Nottingham: NOF, 2004.
- Obesity training courses for primary care (from www.domuk.org)
- Prochaska JO, DiClemente CC, Norcross JC. In search of how people change: applications to addictive behaviours. *Am Psychol* 1992;47:1102-14.
- Scottish Intercollegiate Guidelines Network. Obesity in Scotland: integrating prevention with weight management. www.sign.ac.uk/pdf/sign8.pdf (accessed 12 Jul 2006).
- Counterweight Project Team. A new evidence-based model for weight management in primary care: the Counterweight programme. *J Hum Nutr Diet* 2004;17:191-208.

4 Management: Part II—Drugs

Mike Lean, Nick Finer

Despite the availability of evaluated and approved obesity drugs—and even though some patients will have failed to lose weight after non-drug treatment—doctors have been reluctant to prescribe drugs. The reasons for this may include memories of the adverse events with amphetamine, and amphetamine-like drugs, and the serious complications from combining phentermine and fenfluramine. Current drugs recommended for treating obesity have all been evaluated and approved by regulatory standards that apply to all drug treatments. The use of obesity drugs should follow the principles of any other therapeutic area—that is, they may be prescribed after assessment of the potential benefits and risks (both clinical and economic), with appropriately informed patients, and with medical monitoring of the results of treatment.

Many people, including doctors, still believe that a short course of drug treatment might "cure" obesity or that efficacy is measured only by ever-continuing weight loss. These misconceptions are at odds with biology: people who become obese have a lifelong tendency both to defend their excess weight and to continue to gain extra body fat. Effective management, including drugs when needed, must be life long and focused on weight loss maintenance in a similar fashion to the effective treatment for hypertension or diabetes. Drug efficacy can be considered in terms of the impact on measures such as body mass index or fat distribution, risk factors, disease improvement, or reduction in clinical end points. Starting drug treatment should always be regarded as a therapeutic trial and stopped if weight loss is not apparent after one to two months.

> Diet and exercise play a central role in preventing obesity and are the first line treatment for the condition. But many patients also need drugs to help them lose weight, and to maintain the loss, however that was achieved

Clinical targets from which to evaluate drug efficacy in interventions for weight management

Physical measure	Risk factor	Disease severity	Clinical end points
Changes in mass (body mass loss, maintenance of body mass loss, maintenance of fat loss, body mass index); changes in fat distribution (waist circumference, abdominal fat area,* visceral fat volume†)	High levels of fasting cholesterol and triglycerides; low levels of high density lipoprotein cholesterol; high blood pressure; left ventricular hypertrophy	Glycaemic control; quality of life; left ventricular function	Cardiovascular event; cardiovascular mortality; development of diabetes; unwanted effects; joint pain; sleep apnoea; depression

*Derived from computed tomography or magnetic resonance imaging.
†Predicted from cross sectional computed tomography, magnetic resonance imaging, or (more weakly) dual emission x ray absorptiometry (DEXA)—which measures the density of bones.

Drug treatment of the consequences of obesity

Current approaches to obesity management largely involve trying to treat all the additional symptoms, risk factors for future disease, and existing comorbidity without necessarily tackling the primary problem. The excess polypharmacy administered to obese patients was highlighted in a recent audit of primary care (the UK Counterweight programme).

Obese patients often take five or more different drugs, all for components of metabolic syndrome, plus symptomatic treatments such as use of bronchodilators, analgesics, and drugs for arthritis and angina. Insulin sensitising agents (such as metformin) are sometimes used to try to improve several obesity related risk factors simultaneously, but they rarely adequately improve the hazards and symptoms of obesity, so polypharmacy may still be necessary.

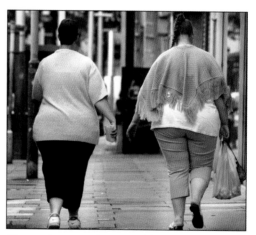

Obese patients are at increased risk from cardiovascular disease: it is imperative that risk factors are treated early and optimally. Effective treatment to prevent the underlying cause (body fat accumulation) would make better clinical and economic sense and is now accepted as a reasonable target for drug development

Treating obesity itself

If the many diseases associated with obesity are causally related, then they will be modified by treatments that can generate weight loss (that is, loss of body fat) and prevent the regain of excess body fat. Inherent in this is a need to establish energy balance at a lower body weight. Temporary weight loss by liposuction does not do this, nor does it affect metabolic risk.

An effective drug against obesity must reduce energy assimilation from food (without compensatory reduction in

> Liposuction removes only subcutaneous fat, which carries little metabolic risk, and energy intake is unaffected; thus body weight will rise again to achieve energy balance

energy expenditure) or stimulate energy expenditure (without compensatory increase in food consumption), or both. Current drugs act mainly on energy intake; for maximal effectiveness, they depend on patients adopting a well designed diet and lifestyle programme. In a recent one year study, intensive lifestyle intervention produced weight loss (6.7 (standard deviation 7.9) kg) similar to that achieved with the drug sibutramine alone (5.0 (7.4) kg); combining lifestyle intervention with the drug doubled the weight loss (12.1 (9.8) kg).

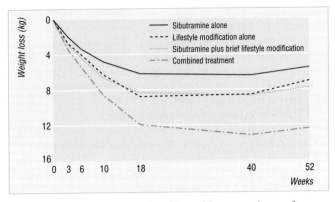

Effects on weight loss of sibutramine with or without some degree of lifestyle modification (adapted from Wadden et al. *N Engl J Med* 2005;353:2111-20)

Principles of drug therapy

Weight loss—The benefit of obesity drugs depends on effects on body fat and body weight. Two thirds of patients can achieve a 5-10% loss in three to six months with lifestyle modification and drug treatment. A weight loss of less than 1-2 kg after six weeks indicates an inadequate response, except in patients who have already lost weight with diet and exercise and patients with type 2 diabetes.

Weight maintenance—Most patients who lose weight regain it. Drugs are a logical treatment not just for weight loss induction but for long term weight loss maintenance. A reasonable long term target is to restrict regain—for example, to below the average rate of weight gain (1-2 kg a year for obese people).

Symptoms and risk factors—Patients should show long term improvements as a consequence of the weight control or through separate mechanisms of the drug.

Duration of treatment—It is logical to continue the drug for as long as it is effective; if the drug is effective, withdrawal will lead to weight regain. Current licensing criteria still limit treatment duration to one to two years, although for some drugs, trials show continuing benefit. Treatment beyond this limit, however, must still be recognised as "off licence," and patients should be counselled and supervised accordingly.

Side effects and safety—Overall risk to benefit of existing drugs has been favourably shown in terms of symptoms, risk factors, and diabetes prevention. As for any other disease, patients have to be seen regularly for benefit to be assessed and unwanted effects identified. Limited information on safety and efficacy exists for elderly people, children, and adolescents. Pregnant and breast feeding women should not take obesity drugs.

Drugs licensed for obesity management

Orlistat

Orlistat is an intestinal lipase inhibitor taken three times daily with meals. It generates malabsorption of 30% of dietary fat. It leads to 5-10% weight loss in 50-60% of patients, and in clinical trials the loss (and related clinical benefit) is largely maintained up to at least four years.

In a recent review by Finer et al (see Further Reading box), when orlistat was compared with placebo, all risk factors for coronary heart disease improved and 37% fewer patients (52% of those with impaired glucose tolerance) developed diabetes over four years. Reduced intestinal fat absorption may have direct effects on improving lipids and insulin sensitivity.

Outcome improved with a structured diet and exercise programme. (A good action plan (known as MAP) is provided, via the makers of orlistat, to patients prescribed the drug.) Patients who do not follow advice to eat a low fat diet (in general < 60 g fat a day) will have steatorrhoea. Gastrointestinal side effects are not necessary for effective weight loss because malabsorption of 20 g of fat is usually asymptomatic and produces an energy deficit of 180 kcal a day.

What current obesity drugs can do

- Increase weight loss by about 4-6 kg beyond what can be achieved by diet alone
- Maintain weight loss (however achieved) 12-15 kg below baseline
- Improve most cardiovascular risks in direct relation to weight loss

Combining drugs with different mechanisms is a logical way to increase efficacy. However, the limited evidence does not support combining orlistat and sibutramine

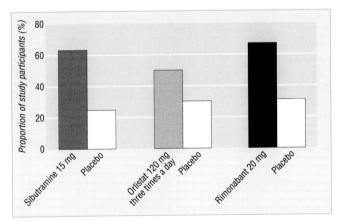

Proportion of study participants achieving 5-10% weight loss in one year, according to drug taken (data from combined datasets of 1 year phase 3 trials of three obesity drugs including rimonabant (adapted from Finer N, see Further Reading box)

Sibutramine

Sibutramine inhibits the reuptake of noradrenaline and serotonin, promoting and prolonging satiety; it is taken once daily. It produces 5-10% weight loss in 60-70% of patients, and in clinical trials it is well maintained for at least two years. If weight loss is less than 2 kg at four weeks, the dose can be increased from 10 mg to 15 mg.

High density lipoprotein cholesterol concentrations increase by 25%, partly independently of weight loss. The noradrenergic action increases heart rate by 1-2 beats/min and attenuates the fall in blood pressure expected with weight loss. Some patients, especially if they fail to lose weight, may record a rise in their blood pressure; it is therefore essential to monitor blood pressure during the first 12 weeks of treatment. Controlled hypertension is not a contraindication for prescribing sibutramine.

Rimonabant

Rimonabant is the first cannabinoid-1 receptor antagonist to be licensed for obesity treatment. Stimulation of cannabinoid-1 receptors in the brain promotes eating and in peripheral tissues cardiovascular risk factors such as low concentration of high density lipoprotein cholesterol, insulin resistance, and inflammation. Blockade with rimonabant produces weight loss and weight-independent improvements of some cardiovascular risk factors.

Rimonabant produces 5-10% weight loss in 60-70% of subjects, maintained for up to two years in clinical trials. Side effects reported were mild and infrequent. Clinical trials excluded depressed patients; effects on mood and depression should be assessed during routine clinical care.

> **The three licensed obesity drugs (orlistat, sibutramine, rimonabant) can all significantly improve glycaemic control in overweight patients with diabetes**

> **Sibutramine's main side effects include a dry mouth, constipation, headaches, and dizziness; all may be improved by drinking more water when losing weight. Poor sleep and agitation may occur early in treatment and are usually self limiting. Several potential drug interactions (for example, with selective serotonin reuptake inhibitors) may limit usage**

Drugs that are not recommended

- Methyl cellulose is still licensed in the UK as an adjunct in obesity, but no evidence exists for its efficacy or safety
- Phentermine is a catecholamine releasing agent that stimulates the central nervous system, producing appetite suppression. Efficacy and safety have not been sufficiently established

Drugs licensed for non-obesity indications

- Any drug that produces anorexia or nausea as a side effect will produce weight loss but would be inappropriate as an obesity treatment.
- Metformin produces minor effects on body weight but improves insulin sensitivity, preventing progression from impaired glucose tolerance to diabetes. It improves fertility in women with polycsytic ovarian syndrome. Gastrointestinal side effects, however, may limit its use.
- In epileptic patients, topiramate (atypical anticonvulsant) produces less weight gain than other anticonvulsants and often striking weight loss. It was withdrawn during clinical trials for use in obesity because of cognitive side effects at effective doses in non-epileptic subjects

---

Incidence of side effects expressed as ratio of active treatment to placebo from clinical trials of orlistat, sibutramine and rimonabant. Adapted from Greenway and Caruso (see Further Reading box)

Symptom	Orlistat	Sibutramine	Rimonabant (20 mg)
Dry mouth	-	4.1	-
Dizziness	1.0	2.4	1.8
Nausea	1.1	2.1	3.0
Diarrhoea	-	-	2.4
Constipation	-	1.9	-
Oily spotting*	20.5	-	-
Flatus with discharge*	20.9	-	-
Faecal urgency*	3.3	-	-
Fatty or oily stool*	6.9	-	-
Oily evacuation*	14.9	-	-
Increased defecation*	2.6	-	-
Faecal incontinence*	8.6	-	-
Musculoskeletal disorder	2.0	1.6	1.1
Anxiety	1.6	1.3	3.3
Depression	0	1.7	12.3
Insomnia	1.2	2.4	
Cardiovascular disorder	1.0	2.2	0.8
Hypertension	-	2.3	-
Tachycardia	-	4.3	-
Palpitation	-	2.5	-

Dashes indicate "not reported."
*These effects occur only if excess fats are eaten.

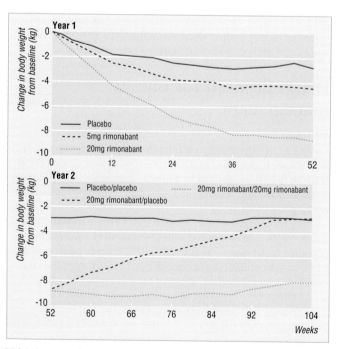

Weight loss over first year of treatment with rimonabant (combined with lifestyle modification) is maintained in year 2 if drug is continued. Weight regain occurs if drug is withdrawn even if lifestyle modification is continued (adapted from Pi-Sunyer et al. *JAMA* 2006;295:761-75)

New drugs in development

Clinical trials are now well advanced for several drugs with different modes of action.

Many of the hormones and hormone receptors that contribute to regulation of appetite or satiety are targets for drug treatment and under active development in preclinical and early clinical trials. Newer agents primarily designed to treat diabetes, such as the synthetic amylin pramlintide and GLP-1 analogue exenatide, are licensed in the US and unlike most other hypoglycaemic drugs lead to clinically important weight loss.

For the very rare cases of leptin deficiency, daily injections are curative. Most obese people, however, have high concentrations of leptin, and trials of hyperaugmentation were disappointing. Rosenbaum et al found that after 10% weight loss induced by a low energy liquid diet, recombinant leptin restored circulating leptin concentrations, energy expenditure, the work efficiency of skeletal muscle, sympathetic nervous system tone, and circulating concentrations of thyroxine and triiodothyronine to levels present before the weight loss (*Journal of Clinical Investigation* 2005;115:3579-86).

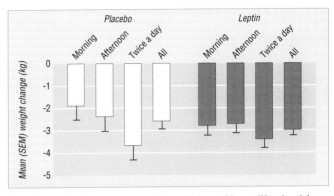

Recombinant leptin given once or twice daily in addition to lifestyle advice on weight loss over 12 weeks in obese subjects with normal plasma leptin concentration shows no benefit over placebo. (Adapted from Zelissen et al. *Diabetes Obes Metab* 2005;7:755-61)

Pharmacoeconomics

Drug treatment is considered effective (in terms of numbers needed to treat) and cost effective by the National Institute for Health and Clinical Excellence, with an overall cost per quality adjusted life year of £19 000 (€27 500; $35 000) to £55 000, which can be further improved by targeting patients with comorbidities.

Cost effectiveness is estimated to vary between €3462 per life year gained for obese diabetic patients with hypertension and hypercholesterolaemia and €19 986 per life year gained for obese diabetic patients without other risk factors (*Diabetes Care* 2002;25:303-8).

Evaluation of drug treatment in routine clinical practice, including cost effectiveness studies, is confounded when data from randomised controlled trials are used because patients who fail to respond to treatment continue to be included. In routine practice, such patients' treatment would be stopped at an early stage. Long term randomised controlled trials of obesity drugs thus tend to exaggerate costs of effective treatment by about 20%.

> Obesity is associated both directly and indirectly (through its comorbidities and excess prescribing) with excess health costs. Effective early treatment with long term weight maintenance may be cost effective

Key references and further reading

- Finer N. Does pharmacologically-induced weight loss improve cardiovascular outcome? Impact of anti-obesity agents on cardiovascular risk. *Eur Heart J Supplements* 2005;7(suppl):L32-8.
- Greenway FL, Caruso MK. Safety of obesity drugs. *Expert Opin Drug Saf* 2005;4(6):1083-95.
- Pagotto U, Vicennati V, Pasquali R. The endocannabinoid system and the treatment of obesity. *Ann Med* 2005;37:270-5.
- Small CJ, Parkinson JR, Bloom SR. Novel therapeutic targets for appetite regulation. *Curr Opinion Invest Drugs* 2005;6:369-72.
- Curran MP, Scott LJ. Orlistat: a review of its use in the management of patients with obesity. *Drugs* 2004;64:2845-64.
- Rissanen A, Lean M, Rossner S, Segal KR, Sjostrom L. Predictive value of early weight loss in obesity management with orlistat: an evidence-based assessment of prescribing guidelines. *Int J Obes Relat Metab Disord* 2003 Jan;27:103-9.

Useful websites

- www.counterweight.org (multicentre obesity management project led by practice nurses, conducted in seven UK regions)
- www.changeforlifeonline.com (week by week plan for lifestyle changes for patients taking sibutramine)
- www.itswhatyougain.co.uk (support site for patients taking rimonabant)
- www.rcplondon.ac.uk/pubs/wp_antiobesitydrugs.htm (Royal College of Physicians' guidelines) (accessed 10 Jul 2006)
- www.nice.org.uk (National Institute for Health and Clinical Excellence is an independent organisation responsible for providing national guidance on promoting good health and preventing and treating ill health)
- www.cochrane.org (for Cochrane reviews)
- www.jr2.ox.ac.uk/bandolier/band100/b100-4.html (for research information on obesity drugs)
- www.obesity-news.com (for research information about obesity drugs)

The photograph at the start of this article is published with permission from Rex.

Competing interests: Nick Finer has received research grants and consultancy fees from, and served on advisory boards to, many pharmaceutical companies involved in the development of treatments for obesity and diabetes, including Roche, Abbott, Sanofi-Aventis, Merck, Shionogi, Pfizer and GlaxoSmithKline.

5 Management: Part III–Surgery

John G Kral

Although surgery can be a potentially life extending treatment for obesity, most patients and doctors reject surgical intervention. Moreover, no national health budget or insurance can afford surgery on a very large scale. However, obesity surgery is a successful, validated, legitimate treatment and needs to be considered in some circumstances.

Preventive surgery

Healthcare workers and the public alike still lack awareness about the epidemiological consequences of and the severity of outcomes associated with pregnancy in obese women. Outcomes include fetal loss, malformations, intellectual impairment, lifelong psychosocial suffering, and programming of chronic metabolic diseases. People also lack awareness about the epigenetic transmission of obesity to their daughters, who themselves go on to become obese mothers.

Given the seriousness of the obesity epidemic, "preventive surgery" in obese young women may therefore be indicated when all else fails. Furthermore, such surgery can prevent the inexorable progression of obesity towards manifest comorbidity (such as diabetes, congestive heart failure, liver cirrhosis, and hypertension) and, ultimately, irreversible chronic disease and end organ failure.

Obesity surgery entails a trade-off between the progressively debilitating intractable symptoms and chronic diseases associated with obesity and the side effects and complications of operations designed to create chronic (relative) undernutrition. Most obese adults who have chosen surgery and had complications (including death) have been satisfied with their choice because their lives as obese individuals were often not worth living.

Early obesity surgery can bring secondary health problems. Nevertheless, the extraordinary lifelong suffering imposed by the psychosocial sequelae of extreme childhood obesity cannot be underestimated: depression, anxiety, eating disorders, vocational and marital failure, and years of life lost. Mitigating the impairment of quality of life might well be the most important outcome measure used to evaluate treatments for childhood obesity. Thus, even surgery can be considered.

Behavioural surgery

The different types of operations (restrictive versus bypass) have different and substantive long term effects on eating (the most important of all activities of daily living)—thus the term "behavioural surgery."

Prerequisites for considering obesity surgery are extensive patient assessment and meticulous preoperative education. Identifying motivational factors driving the patient to maintain obesity is more important before surgery than before non-surgical treatments because of the greater stakes involved.

"Successful" surgery has more potential for achieving meaningful, durable weight loss, and "failure" after surgery has much graver consequences. Assessment and education should allow improved allocation of patients to specific types of operations and postoperative care.

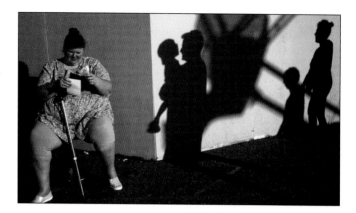

Without understanding or accepting the severity of obesity and the risks of obesity (or "bariatric") surgery—or the "success" and risks of non-surgical alternatives—doctors and other health workers cannot adequately advise patients in their choice of treatment

Compared with usual care, obesity surgery has recently been shown to reduce all cause mortality, mortality due to cancer, and cardiovascular mortality

---

Goal and methods of obesity surgery

Goal

To prevent or reduce storage of excess energy as fat

Methods

Physical—To reduce energy intake and absorption and to increase energy output

Appetite—To increase satiety (pleasant sense of fullness) or neutrality (neither hunger nor fullness); or to increase nimiety (unpleasant feeling of fullness) through aversion and discomfort

---

Key prerequisites for obesity surgery

- Assessment of the patient to uncover motivational factors
- Comprehensive, preoperative education for the patient
- A team experienced in bariatric laparoscopic surgery

16

Obstructive and diversionary operations

As with most surgery, bariatric surgery should preferably be performed laparoscopically and only by surgeons with sufficient training and expertise. Surgeon and hospital case volume affect perioperative safety: the more cases, the better the outcomes. Because of the adverse interaction between obesity and inflammatory and physiological processes related to incision size and an open abdomen, obese patients benefit more from laparoscopic approaches than other patients, regardless of operation or condition being treated.

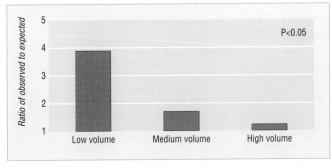

Ratio of observed to expected inhospital mortality for patients aged ≥55 years, according to bariatric surgical volume (adapted from Nguyen et al. *Ann Surg* 2004;240:586-94)

The simplest operation is laparoscopic placement of an inflatable band encircling the top 5% of the stomach, creating a proximal "pouch." During follow-up a physician can inject or withdraw saline to adjust the diameter of the band, which obstructs or restricts the passage of mainly solids (high energy liquids readily pass through). Discomfort or involuntary vomiting, or both, occur after poor chewing (such as from ill fitting dentures), rapid eating, exceeding pouch capacity (about 20 ml), or drinking shortly after eating. Repeated vomiting may cause the pouch to stretch, allowing weight gain.

Complex laparoscopic operations combine obstruction and diversion (or bypass), disconnecting the proximal pouch from the stomach and attaching it to a limb of the small bowel (known as the Roux-en-Y gastric bypass). Variations of gastric bypass—such as the biliopancreatic diversion and long limb gastric bypass, which leave less absorptive small bowel in continuity—are reserved for heavier patients with more intractable disease and severe binge eating disorder. Heavier patients (with a very high body mass index—calculated as dividing the weight in kilograms by the height in metres squared) have binge eating disorder.

Outcomes of 24 166 patients having obesity surgery in 93 US academic hospitals by volume, 1992-2002

	High volume (>100 cases/year)	Medium volume (50-100 cases/year)	Low volume (<50 cases/year)
Mean No of cases/year	157	71	15
Mean No of days of stay	3.8*	4.4	5.1*
Mortality (%)	0.3*	0.5	1.2*
Complications (all types) (%)	10.2*	12.3	14.5*
Complications of medical care (%)	7.8*	9.5	10.8*

*P < 0.05. Data from Nguyen et al. *Ann Surg* 2004;240:586-94.

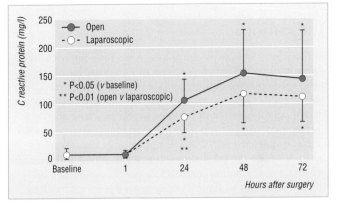

Inflammatory response (C reactive protein) to open *v* laparoscopic gastric bypass (adapted from Nguyen et al. *J Am Coll Surg* 2002;194:562)

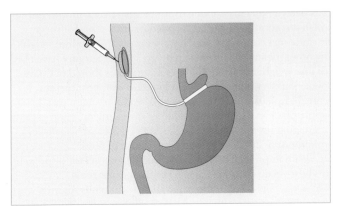

Adjustable gastric band showing injection or withdrawal of saline to adjust diameter of band

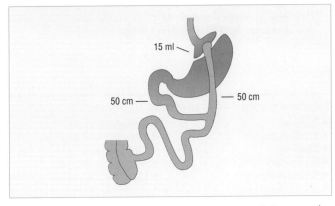

Roux-en-Y gastric bypass with pouch separated from stomach (laparoscopic technique)

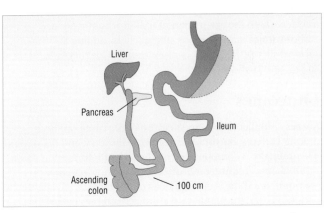

Biliopancreatic diversion with sleeve resection of greater curvature and post-pyloric, duodeno-ileal anastomosis ("duodenal switch")

17

During the first eight to 12 months after bypass operations, weight loss is caused by obstruction of nutrient flow. After the stomach pouch and its enterostomy stretch, continued and maintained weight loss is caused partly by altered processing and/or absorption of nutrients and partly by decreased appetite or "hunger" owing to the rush of nutrients into the limb of the small bowel.

The generic types of operations have different effects on eating behaviour, the key element of obesity, so results, risks, and benefits can vary substantially. Obstructive operations require frequent outpatient visits (monthly during the first 12-18 months) to optimise weight loss. Diversionary operations (requiring clinic visits every three months during the first year) consistently achieve greater and better maintained weight loss than gastric banding. Their greater risk of long term complications is abrogated by one yearly clinic visit with blood testing for vitamin and mineral deficiencies.

Indications

Both surgical and non-surgical treatments have improved over the past 25 years. Diet and exercise programmes have been developed and four new drugs have been launched. The safety and efficacy of surgery has improved remarkably. Calculations of cost per kilogram of maintained weight loss have shown a "break even" comparison after less than four years—results that favour surgery, if costs of drugs, supplements, complications and side effects are taken into account. For ethical and scientific reasons, randomisation studies of surgery and non-surgical treatment cannot be done. Furthermore, it is very difficult to retain participants in non-surgical treatment long enough to provide meaningful comparable outcome data.

The widely accepted indication for surgery since the 1960s has been a body mass index (BMI) of ≥ 40 or 35-40 with obesity related comorbidity. Recommended requirements for surgery include that patients should have seriously tried to lose weight by other means. In fact, most patients seeking surgery have tried to lose weight five to seven times. Candidates should not have behavioural conditions likely to interfere with postoperative care. Hospitals should have a multidisciplinary team with appropriate expertise for evaluating, operating on, and managing severely obese patients. Age criteria are usually a minimum of 20-25 years and a maximum of 60-65.

With improved safety—owing to the laparoscopic approach and the relatively simple and reversible gastric band technique—indications are expanding, with trends towards accepting patients with a lower BMI (30-35) and a wider age range (from adolescence (12-17 years) to 70 years and above) in appropriate candidates. Weight regain after purely restrictive operations can be treated by using "rescue" medication (which interferes with the absorption of lipids (orlistat) and/or carbohydrates (acarbose)) or, ultimately, by adding a diversionary procedure.

Outcomes

Success is difficult to define because of disparate opinions among patients, doctors, the insurance industry, and tax payers. The difficulty is compounded by the lack of information about optimal amounts and rates of weight loss: how much is "enough" and how is enough determined? Actuarial data define "desirable" weight standards for the general population, but insufficient and conflicting data are available for those who have lost weight voluntarily and maintained the loss.

Mechanisms of obesity surgery

Procedures that are only obstructive
- Delayed emptying of solids
- Diminished capacity for solids
- Oesophagogastric distension

Bypass procedures
- Transitory restriction
- Altered absorption
- Neuroendocrine effects on appetite

Instructions on eating for patients who have had obstructive stomach surgery

Eating and drinking	Vomiting
Eat slowly and undisturbed	If you vomit, find out why
Chew well	Don't eat or drink for four hours
Drink before food or more than an hour after food	Start with liquids after four hours
Stop if your stomach feels full	If you still vomit, call your surgeon

---

Indications for obesity surgery must be viewed in the context of results of alternative, non-surgical treatments and their costs and risks, and the patient's assessment of quality of life. This supports the importance of educating and assessing patients. Data showing superior efficacy of obesity surgery over optimal non-surgical treatment have been unequivocal since the early 1960s, when such surgery began

---

Suitability for referral for surgery
- Candidates should understand the medical need to lose weight and have previously tried to lose weight
- They should have no psychological or psychiatric problems that might interfere with follow-up (drug misuse, borderline personality)
- There should be sufficient resources for follow-up (a multidisciplinary team, compassionate partner, and time)

High risk patients, especially men with a BMI of >55, need complex surgery and may benefit from a staged approach, starting with a simple restrictive operation, followed as needed (depending on weight loss maintenance) by a diversionary stage

---

Conditions improved or prevented by obesity
- Asthma
- Cancers (many)
- Diabetes
- Dyslipidaemia
- Oesophagitis
- Heart failure
- Hypertension
- Infectious diseases
- Infertility surgery
- Obstetric complications
- Operative risk
- Liver cirrhosis
- Quality of life
- Sleep apnoea
- Thrombosis

Rather than focusing on weight loss as the primary outcome measure, it is more appropriate to evaluate improvements in comorbidities and quality of life, although in patients with a BMI of >35 mortality (including operative) is lower in patients having operations than in those receiving usual care. Numerous observational and case studies over four decades have consistently found improved established risk factors for premature death, reduction of comorbidity, and improved quality of life after surgical weight loss.

At the same time, obesity surgery is associated with mortality, morbidity, complications, side effects, and unwanted sequelae, all of which must be included in the risk-benefit analysis. Mortality statistics need stratification by generic type of operation, age, sex, and comorbidity profile. However, it is difficult preoperatively to predict long term outcomes for the various types of operations. Social factors such as having a stable life situation (being married, having a job) and being white predict favourable outcomes, whereas binge eating or overconsumption of "soft calories" (calories derived from liquids or soft foods such as ice cream and chocolate) may be detrimental.

Deficiencies of vitamins and minerals are among the most common and troublesome long term complications of obesity surgery. They are more common after diversionary operations, due to poor digestion and malabsorption from exclusion of the stomach and shortened continuous small bowel. Vitamin and mineral deficiency is preventable with assiduous monitoring and adequate supplementation, both of which require the patient's cooperation, which often is difficult to achieve.

As with all surgery, the proficiency and dedication of the surgeons and their teams are critical. Obesity surgery has become the victim of its own success owing to improved perioperative results, general awareness of the seriousness of the disease, and substantial increases in the numbers of obese patients, which has led to the rapid recruitment of surgeons who are not yet sufficiently trained. Currently, strict guidelines and performance evaluations are being developed as part of quality assurance efforts and demands from third party payers.

Conclusions

- Operations use different mechanisms for weight loss
- One type of operation does not fit all
- Preoperative evaluation and patient education are critical
- The laparoscopic approach is preferable
- Surgery reduces mortality compared with usual care

Further reading

- Christou NV, Sampalis JS, Liberman M, Look D, Auger S, McLean AP, et al. Surgery decreases long term mortality, morbidity and healthcare use in morbidly obese patients. *Ann Surg* 2004;240:416-24.
- Sjöström L, Lindroos AK, Peltonen M, Torgerson J, Bouchard C, Carlsson B, et al. Lifestyle, diabetes, and cardiovascular risk factors 10 years after bariatric surgery. *N Engl J Med* 2004;351:2683-93.
- Sugerman HG, Kral JG. Evidence-based medicine reports on bariatric surgery: a critique. *Int J Obes* 2005;29:735-45.
- Kral JG. Preventing and treating obesity in girls and young women to curb the epidemic. *Obes Res* 2004;12:1539-46.
- Livingston EH, Martin RF, eds. Bariatric surgery. *Surg Clin N Am* 2005;85(4):665-874.
- Sjöström L. Soft and hard endpoints over 5-18 years in the intervention trial Swedish obese subjects. *Obesity Reviews* 2006;7(suppl 2):27.

The photograph is published with permission from Constantine Manos/Magnum Photos.

Adverse effects of obesity surgery

Operative (about 10%)	Long term (20-30%)
Thromboembolism	Iron deficiency
Bleeding	Calcium and vitamin D deficiency
Pneumonia	Vitamin B-12 deficiency
Stenosis	Vitamin B-1 deficiency (vomiting)
Ulcers	Protein deficiency (diarrhoea)
Infection or hernia	Gallstones
Peritonitis	Weight regain
Death ≤ 1%	

Predictors of response

Demographic—Age, sex, race, marital status, education, job, insurance

Physiological—Body mass index, body composition (fat cell size, fat distribution, lean body mass), metabolic rate (resting, total, diet*), blood chemistry

Comorbidity—Diabetes, hypertension, cardiopulmonary disease, sleep apnoea, musculoskeletal disorders, thromboembolism

Psychological—MMPI disorder,† sexual abuse, negative life experience, secondary gain, codependency, denial of disease

Past performance—Weight loss, smoking cessation, attendance at appointments, drug and alcohol use

Eating behaviour—Eating sweets, nibbling, gorging, binge eating, restrained eating, poor impulse control

*Diet induced thermogenesis.
†According to Minnesota multiphasic personality inventory

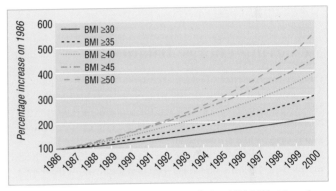

Obesity trends in United States, by body mass index, 1986-2000. Adapted from Sturm R. *Arch Intern Med* 2003;163: 2146-8

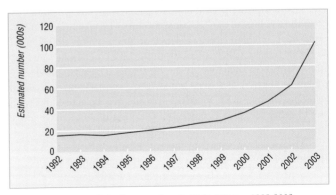

Estimated numbers of obesity operations in United States, 1992-2003. Adapted from Steinbrook R. *N Engl J Med* 2004;350:1075-9

Competing interests: John G Kral is a member of the North American Association for the Study of Obesity and the American Society for Bariatric Surgery.

6 Strategies for preventing obesity

Mike Lean, Jose Lara, James O Hill

Obesity is an epidemic, says the World Health Organization. The prevalence of adult obesity has exceeded 30% in the United States, is over 20% in most of Europe (5-23% in men, 7-36% in women), and is 40-70% in the Gulf states and Polynesian islands. Obesity is also present in low income countries, and low socioeconomic groups are affected most. In most countries the prevalence of obesity now exceeds 15%, the figure used by WHO to define the critical threshold for intervention in nutritional epidemics.

Obese people are at high risk of multiple health problems and need full medical management. The numbers are so great (and rising), however, that individual medical care becomes impractical and prohibitively expensive. Currently, the cost of obesity to a country's health service is estimated at up to 9%, and the overall social cost of the condition is seen as a major hindrance to economic development. An even larger proportion of the population is overweight, with increased morbidity. Virtually all the costs (personal, health, and economic) of obesity are met in adulthood and result from fat that has accumulated in adulthood, but there is a likely additional cost due to inactivity and overweight in childhood that should also be considered.

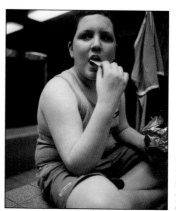

Obesity is increasingly affecting younger people, with warning signs for the future from the increasing prevalence of overweight in childhood

There seems to be strong biological resistance to weight loss once obesity is established. The long term solution must now include effective prevention directed at the whole population

Achieving energy balance

Obesity is a disorder of energy balance ("energy in" equals "energy out"). Weight is steady when energy is balanced. "Positive energy balance" is when the amount of energy consumed as food and drink exceeds the energy used. UK adults on average consume 20 kcal a day more than they expend, leading to an average weight gain of 1 kg a year. Some people who become obese eat 100 kcal a day more than they expend so gain up to 5 kg a year. Any intervention that changes positive energy balance will ultimately be effective in preventing calorie accumulation, thus accumulation of body fat.

The components amenable to intervention are physical activity and overall energy consumption. The absolute level (in kcal/day), at which energy balance occurs is mainly determined by body weight, which affects both the basal metabolic rate and the energy cost of activity. It can be changed by substantial changes in physical activity but also, to a similar degree, by small changes in weight. So some thin people may be active and eat a lot to achieve energy balance, but overweight people have to eat more than most thin people to avoid weight loss.

This purely mechanistic approach cannot be used for health promotion without a fuller understanding of several elements: the balance between individual and genetic predisposition to weight gain; the psychological, social, cultural, and economic and political components of our "obesogenic" environment; and the nature of the "disease vectors" (high energy foods and energy saving devices). Changes in diet and physical activity are necessary for weight loss but do not guarantee it. To avoid compensation (between changes in physical activity and changes in appetite), effective interventions must tackle both diet and physical activity, and in an integrated way.

Differences between individual and population based approaches to obesity. Adapted from Swinburn et al (see Further Reading box)

	Individual based approach	Population based approach
Key measures	Body weight, waist, body mass index	Prevalence of overweight and obesity, mean body mass index, mean waist
Key aetiology question	Why is this person obese (or gaining weight)?	Why does this population have a high (or rising) prevalence of obesity?
Main aetiological mechanisms	Genetic, metabolic, hormonal, behavioural	Environmental, cultural, behavioural
Key management question	What are the best long term strategies for reducing the person's body fat?	What are the best long term strategies for reducing the population's mean body fat/waist circumference?
Main management actions	Patient education, behavioural modification, drugs, surgery	Public education, improving food, physical activity environments, policy, planning
Volume of information on aetiology and management	Vast	Minimal
Driving forces for research and action	Immediate and powerful	Distant and weak
Potential for long term benefit to individuals	Modest	Modest
Potential for long-term benefit to populations	Modest	Significant
Sustainability	Poor	High

A successful intervention for obesity prevention must influence energy balance but must also be sustainable. Changes in diet and physical activity need to be incorporated into new behaviour patterns, as a need for constant reminders or rewards will result in non-sustainability.

A permanent change in the environment is the best way to ensure permanent changes. Actions should focus on (a) enabling people to manage energy balance better in the current environment; (b) modifying the vectors of obesity; and (c) changing the current sociopolitical environment, which currently rewards the manufacturers of products and processes that contribute to obesity. Effective programmes for obesity prevention probably encourage both healthy eating and physical activity (rather than rely on separate strategies for eating and activity).

Strategies that work

Less than 30% of all people in Western countries avoid becoming overweight and maintain a body mass index of <25 throughout their adult life. Among this group, many avoid weight gain only by conscious efforts. Of the 75% of all people who will become overweight, about half will become obese. Thus probably about half of all adults are consciously avoiding further weight gain and have a body mass index of <30. Precisely how they do this is uncertain because of systematic errors in survey methods.

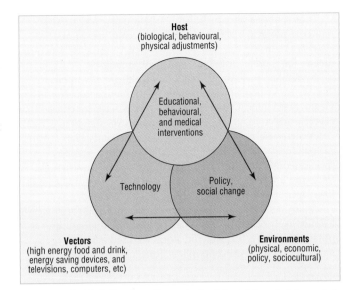

Epidemiological "triad" as it applies to obesity. Adapted from Swinburn et al (see Further Reading box)

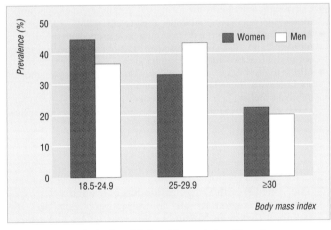

Prevalence of obesity in the adult Scottish population. These figures combine all ages. Among older people, only a quarter to a third remain in the desirable weight range. Data from Scottish health survey, 1998 (www.show.scot.nhs.uk/scottishhealthsurvey/sh8-00.html)

Participants in the US National Weight Control Registry who have successfully lost an average of 30 kg and maintained that loss report high levels of physical activity, equivalent to about an hour a day of moderate intensity physical activity. Successful "maintainers" also reduce dietary fat intake to a lower level than in the general population.

A recent US telephone survey from the Colorado "On the Move" initiative reports that, on average, individuals of normal weight walk 600 more steps a day than overweight individuals and 2400 more than obese individuals. People aged over 60—particularly widowers, those in low income families, and obese individuals—are the main group who would benefit from increased physical activity. Watching television for over three hours a day is a major barrier to physical activity.

Strategies used by individuals to control weight problems

- Decrease dietary fat consumption
- Skip meals or don't skip meals
- Decrease fizzy drinks or replace them with low sugar drinks
- Avoid sugary foods and processed high-fat meat products
- Increase low energy foods (such as fruits and vegetables)
- Choose natural foods if possible, but if buying manufactured or packaged foods, buy those low in energy density
- Eat off small plates; avoid large portions (never "super size")
- Never eat with fingers
- Only eat when sitting down
- Join a gym
- Use a gym
- Walk to the gym
- Walk more and don't bother with the gym
- Get a pedometer and use it to monitor increased walking

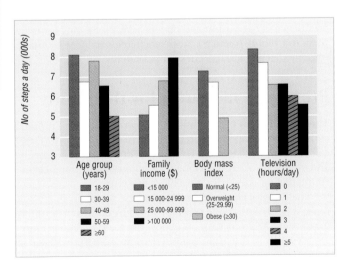

Colorado "On the Move" survey of walking. Data from *Med Sci Sports Exerc* 2005;37:724-30

Combining a low fat diet with exercise is particularly valuable for preventing diabetes and hypertension and is likely to be effective in preventing weight gain

21

Interventions have included increasing physical activity; reducing physical inactivity (usually reducing television viewing); reducing total calories and energy density of foods or dietary fats; and a combination of these strategies.

Systematic reviews by England's Health Development Agency (now incorporated into the National Institute for Health and Clinical Excellence) and others have concluded that exercise added to a diet programme improves weight loss.

A meta-analysis of studies on reducing dietary fats by using normal food or food lower in fat concluded that people spontaneously consumed about 270 kcal a day less when following lower fat diets, effectively resetting energy balance at a lower level, thereby avoiding about 15 kg of weight gain.

Measures successful in preventing weight regain after weight loss are likely to apply in primary prevention. Increasing physical activity is a key factor, along with reducing energy intake. Long term prevention has not yet been demonstrated.

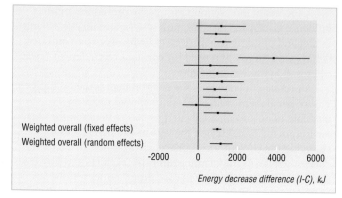

Meta-analysis of role of unrestricted low fat diets in body weight control: differences in energy intake in studies lasting two to 12 months (change in intervention (I) minus change in control (C)) with 95% confidence interval. Adapted from Astrup et al (see Further Reading box)

Small changes can prevent weight gain

The weight gain and current obesity levels in the US population have been shown to result from only a slight shift towards positive energy balance. Thus most weight gain could be prevented with small behavioural changes of this order, such as increased walking, small decreases in dietary fat or sugar intake, and smaller portion sizes. This approach is likely to be more sustainable and effective in preventing weight gain than advocating unnecessary larger changes.

Over 90% of the weight gain seen in US adults results from a positive energy balance of <100 kcal a day

Interventions in children

School based programmes seem promising. They can increase physical activity, particularly in girls, and to a certain extent can modify dietary intake. The effects on weight are not apparent, possibly owing to the short duration of the interventions. Changing the school environment to reduce consumption of high energy food, such as fizzy drinks and foods high in fat and sugar, may help. For example, reducing the consumption of fizzy drinks for 12 months among 7-11 year olds can reduce the prevalence of overweight and obesity by 7.5%. Serving lower fat versions of some popular school lunch items reduces fat intake without affecting attractiveness or palatability.

Childhood overweight and obesity
- Overweight and obesity are increasing in children of all ages, and "obese" teenagers enter adult life already with a BMI >25
- Although obese children do not often have immediate health problems, and most obese adults were not obese as children, many obese children become obese adults
- Efforts to prevent obesity in childhood and its progression into adulthood are fuelled by a belief that it might be possible to influence lifelong behavioural patterns

Preventive measures for the future

The World Health Organization's Regional Office for Europe considers obesity prevention to be one of its highest priorities. It called for immediate, comprehensive action by governments and others in society by arranging a ministerial conference on counteracting obesity for November this year.

The organisation is advocating a range of actions that would make it easier for people to adopt a healthy lifestyle. The aim is to prevent further increase in obesity rates and to reduce rates progressively in the next decade. Given the rising prevalence of obesity, even attenuating the rise should be seen as a success. A further problem for health planners is that obesity and its secondary health costs are associated with more socially deprived and minority population groups. Any measures based on cognitive, educative interventions will tend to benefit more educated and affluent people, thus accentuating the social health gradient. Measures directed at changing the price, availability, and nutritional characteristics of food may have a positive effect across social groups.

The World Health Organization has convened a ministerial conference on "counteracting obesity" in Istanbul, Turkey, in November this year, where a charter on counteracting obesity will be signed

Core actions proposed by WHO
- Reducing commercial pressure on people (particularly children) to consume high energy products
- Reducing fat, sugar, and salt in manufactured products
- Enabling easier and cheaper access to healthy food
- Introducing measures to improve food and increase physical activity in schools and the workplace
- Promoting cycling and walking by better urban design and transport policies
- Creating opportunities in local environments for people to be more physically active in their leisure time
- Encouraging health services to provide advice on diet and physical activity, and promote exclusive breast feeding

WHO has advocated the involvement of the different government sectors, as well as the private sector and civil society. The European Union's initiative the "Platform on Diet and Physical Activity" has stimulated commitments from the food industry and advertisers. The relevance and effectiveness of these commitments is being evaluated. The US private sector has sponsored initiatives such as "America on the Move," which is based on the "small changes" approach.

One scenario includes the reduction of existing obesity. On average, adults now eat 500-600 kcal more than they did 30 years ago, of which 50 kcal a day represent continuing weight gain and about 500 kcal a day maintain current levels of overweight and obesity. If everyone were to eat 500-600 kcal a day less than they currently do, then their weight would fall by 10-30 kg and current obesity levels would reduce to those of 30 years ago. This strategy, however, works for less than 30% of people attending one-to-one obesity clinics and its success on a large scale seems improbable.

The alternative scenario—a "small changes" strategy—is more realistic. This strategy aims to increase physical activity and reduce energy intake both by 100 kcal a day to prevent further weight gain. It accepts that those already overweight and obese will remain so. The next generation is thus the true target for obesity prevention—lifestyle changes would be started in childhood and sustained for life.

The photographs on the first page and this page are published with permission from Gusto/SPL and David Zalubowski/AP/Empics respectively.

Competing interests: James O Hill has served on advisory panels and received consulting fees from PepsiCo, General Mills, GSK Pharmaceuticals, and Slimfast Nutrition. He has received funding from McNeil Nutritionals.

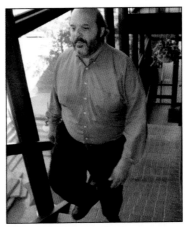

America on the Move uses the principle that increasing the daily number of steps walked by 2000 above current levels (using a pedometer), plus choosing one way to cut out 100 kcal, can prevent weight gain in most children and their parents

Further reading

- Astrup A, Grunwald GK, Melanson EL, Saris WH, Hill JO. The role of low-fat diets in body weight control: a meta-analysis of ad libitum dietary intervention studies. *Int J Obes Relat Metab Disord* 2000;24:1545-52.
- Avenell A, Broom J, Brown TJ, Poobalan A, Aucott L, Stearns SC, et al. Systematic review of the long-term effects and economic consequences of treatments for obesity and implications for health improvement. *Health Technol Assess* 2004;8(21).
- Fogelholm M, Kukkonen-Harjula K. Does physical activity prevent weight gain—a systematic review. *Obes Rev* 2000;1:95-111.
- James J, Thomas P, Cavan D, Kerr D. Preventing childhood obesity by reducing consumption of carbonated drinks: cluster randomised controlled trial. *BMJ* 2004;328:1237-9.
- Swinburn B, Egger G. Preventive strategies against weight gain and obesity. *Obes Rev* 2002;3:289-301.
- World Health Organization. *Obesity: preventing and managing the global epidemic.* Geneva: WHO, 1997. (WHO Technical Report Series, No 894.)
- Rodearmel SJ, Wyatt HR, Barry MJ, Dong F, Pan D, Israel RG, et al. A family-based approach to preventing excessive weight gain. *Obesity* 2006;14:1392-401.

7 Risk factors for diabetes and coronary heart disease

Sarah H Wild, Christopher D Byrne

Diabetes

Many cross sectional and prospective studies have confirmed the association between obesity and type 2 diabetes. Most people with type 2 diabetes are overweight or obese: more than 85% of people with type 2 diabetes in southeast Scotland in 2005 had a body mass index (weight in kilograms divided by height in metres squared) of over 25. Recent evidence indicates that high waist circumference may be an even better indicator than body mass index (BMI) of increased risk of type 2 diabetes.

The risk of developing diabetes over a 14 year follow-up period (among nurses aged 30-55 years at baseline) in the nurses' health study was 49 times higher among women whose baseline BMI was >35 than among women whose baseline BMI was <22. Even a slightly raised BMI (22.0-22.9) at follow-up was associated with an age adjusted relative risk of diabetes that was three times higher than that in women with a BMI of <22.0 at follow-up.

Similar findings have been reported for men from a United States cohort of 51 529 male health professionals aged 40-75 in 1986 who were followed until 1992. Those with a BMI of ≥35 had a relative risk of developing diabetes of 42 (95% confidence interval 22.0-80.6) compared with men with a BMI of <23.0 at age 21, after adjustment for age, smoking, and family history of diabetes. Moreover, earlier onset of type 2 diabetes is associated with a higher BMI, and increasing prevalence of overweight and obesity is the most important factor in the increasing number of younger people diagnosed with type 2 diabetes.

These data have been derived from mainly white populations, and ethnicity modifies the relation between BMI and risk of diabetes. In an Indian population the increasing risk of diabetes associated with increasing BMI starts at even lower BMI levels (15 to 20) than in most other ethnic groups (in whom increasing prevalence of diabetes is only observed at a BMI of >25). This difference is only partly explained by patterns of fat distribution in different ethnic groups; south Asian populations are more likely to have a greater total percentage of body fat mass and larger amount of abdominal fat (reflected by high waist circumference) than other ethnic groups at a given level of BMI. High waist circumference increases the risk of glucose intolerance and diabetes, independent of the risk reflected by high BMI.

Studies in China, the US, and Finland have shown that diabetes can be prevented or delayed in people at high risk of diabetes through a combination of change in diet and lifestyle and modest weight loss. In the Swedish obesity study 69% of people with diabetes at baseline who lost weight after gastric bypass surgery did not have diabetes two years after follow-up. The challenges of maintaining weight loss and improvements in health among people with type 2 diabetes are summarised in Cochrane reviews of non-pharmacological and pharmacological interventions (see earlier article in this series).

Hypertension

Blood pressure increases with increasing BMI. The health survey for England 2003 found that mean systolic blood

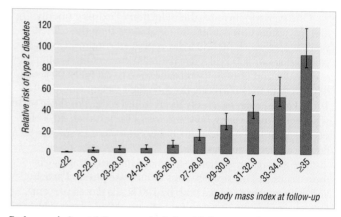

Body mass index at follow-up and relative risk for type 2 diabetes in participants in nurses' health study. Data derived from Colditz et al (see Further Reading box)

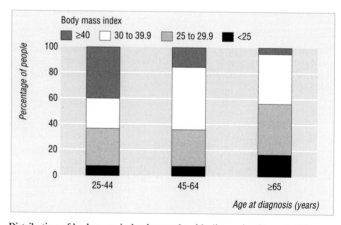

Distribution of body mass index in people with diagnosis of type 2 diabetes in past two years, by age at diagnosis (based on 371, 1466, 1302 people aged 25-44, 45-64, and ≥65 respectively at diagnosis, in population based diabetes register in Lothian, Scotland)

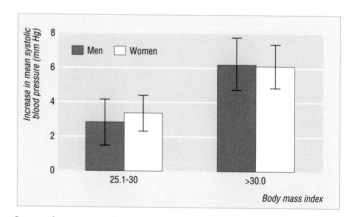

Increase in mean systolic blood pressure in overweight and obese men and women compared with normal weight individuals. Data from *Health Survey for England, 2003* (www.dh.gov.uk)

pressure was about 6 mm Hg higher in obese men and women than in those of normal weight (BMI 18.5-25).

According to data from the third national health and nutrition examination survey (NHANES III) in the US, high blood pressure was the most common condition related to overweight and obesity that showed a marked increase with increasing categories of BMI. The prevalence of high blood pressure (defined as a doctor's diagnosis of hypertension or high blood pressure, or a mean of three readings of > 140 mm Hg for systolic and > 90 mm Hg for diastolic blood pressure) was 2.5 times higher in men and over three times higher in women aged < 55 whose BMI was 30-34.9 than in people of the same age whose BMI was 18.5-24.9. Among people aged ≥ 55, the excess risk of hypertension was less marked for obese people compared with the normal weight group.

Prevalence of hypertension (as defined above) rose from 15% for the normal weight category for both men and women to 42% among obese men and 38% among obese women. Age adjusted prevalence of hypertension was higher among black than white people in each BMI category for both sexes.

These data from NHANES III show that the effect of obesity on risk of hypertension differs with age (higher relative risk among younger age groups but higher absolute risk among older age groups) and ethnicity (higher risk among black than white populations).

Evidence from both American and British populations suggests a stronger relation between blood pressure and central obesity than between blood pressure and peripheral or general fat distribution. Systolic blood pressure was found to increase in a linear manner across the whole range of waist to hip ratio, independently of age, BMI, and other covariates in 9936 men and 12 154 women aged 45-79 years who took part in the Norfolk component of the European Prospective Investigation into Cancer and Nutrition (EPIC-Norfolk). These data were obtained from cross sectional studies, but the clear relation between obesity and subsequent hypertension has also been shown in prospective studies. Interpreting the results of cross sectional studies can be difficult because of potential bias.

Dyslipidaemia

Obesity is associated with both higher levels of total cholesterol and an unfavourable lipid pattern, with low concentrations of HDL (high density lipoprotein) cholesterol and high triglyceride concentrations. This dyslipidaemic pattern is particularly marked in people with central obesity.

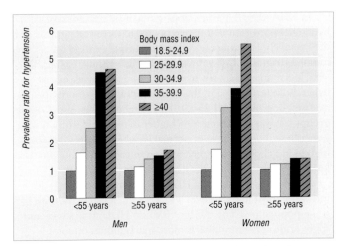

Prevalence ratios for hypertension (that is, a doctor's diagnosis or three readings of ≥140/90 mm Hg) by sex, age, and BMI category. Data derived from cross sectional data from the NHANES III study (Must et al (see Further Reading box))

Weight gain and hypertension

● Weight gain is associated with an increased risk of developing hypertension, but "weight cycling" (repeated gain and loss of weight) does not seem to be

● Long term reductions in blood pressure and reduced risk of hypertension have been achieved with modest weight loss among people aged 30 to 54 who were overweight and had high normal blood pressure levels at baseline

● The number of drugs required to control blood pressure has been shown to be lower among people in a weight loss intervention group

Some of the effect of obesity on blood pressure may be permanent: one study found that blood pressure decreased initially after gastric surgery but after eight years the prevalence of hypertension had returned to the preoperative level

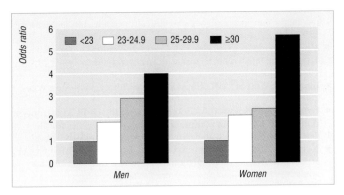

Odds ratios for hypertriglyceridaemia (triglycerides >1.7 mmol/l) by sex and BMI category. Data derived from cross sectional study of 6318 Taiwanese (3540 men, 2778 women) attending health screening centres in southern Taiwan in 2002-3 (Tsai et al. *Am J Epidemiol* 2004;160:557-65)

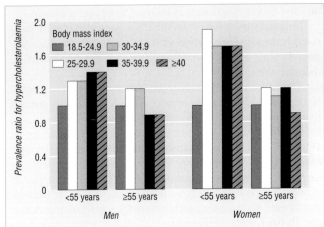

Prevalence ratios for hypercholesterolaemia (that is, a doctor's diagnosis or a measurement of ≥6.2 mmol/l) by sex, age, and BMI category. Data derived from cross sectional data from the NHANES III study (Must et al (see Further Reading box))

In NHANES III, participants were considered to have hypercholesterolaemia if they reported a doctor's diagnosis or if their total cholesterol concentration was higher than 6.2 mmol/l. Trends in hypercholesterolaemia with increasing BMI were less marked than for hypertension. The prevalence of hypercholesterolaemia in this study was highest among the overweight group (BMI 25-29.9) and slightly lower in the obese groups but was still about 50% higher in men and women who were obese than in those of normal weight. The prevalence of high blood cholesterol concentration in each BMI category was lower in black and Hispanic than in white populations.

Mean concentrations of HDL cholesterol decreased with increasing BMI in both sexes and were higher in black than in white populations. The effect of BMI on HDL cholesterol and triglyceride concentrations is more marked than on total cholesterol. The association of waist circumference with lipids and novel markers of lipid associated risk (such as apolipoprotein B or lipoprotein subfractions) is at least as good as that between BMI and lipids.

Smoking

The relation between obesity and smoking is complex: smoking is associated with lower BMI; smoking cessation is linked with weight gain. In many developed countries, however, smoking and obesity are generally associated with lower socioeconomic status and often occur together. Studies examining the effects of BMI that do not take into account smoking habit may be biased and underestimate the harmful effects of increasing BMI.

In addition, smoking seems to be associated with an altered pattern of fat distribution and increased waist circumference. A cross sectional study of Dutch women showed that BMI decreased but that waist to hip ratio increased with increasing number of cigarettes smoked per day. The EPIC-Norfolk study also collected lifestyle data using questionnaires and anthropometric measurements. Current smokers had the highest waist to hip ratios and "never smokers" had the lowest waist to hip ratios after adjustment for age, BMI, alcohol intake, total energy intake, physical activity, and education.

A study of trends in obesity in Texas found that, although smoking cessation was associated with weight gain, the contribution of smoking cessation to trends in overweight and obesity was small. The benefits of smoking cessation may be partly offset by weight gain, although, at least in women, this may not be associated with an increase in fat accumulation.

National survey data from the US suggest that obesity has roughly the same association with chronic health conditions as does 20 years of ageing and that this is considerably greater than the effect of smoking.

The effect of obesity on hospital costs and drug use (36% increase and 77% increase respectively) is considerably greater than for smoking (21% increase and 28% increase respectively).

The National Audit Office estimated that in England in 1998, 10% of deaths were attributable to smoking and 6% to obesity. As smoking levels decline and prevalence of obesity increases, the relative importance of these factors will probably change. A recent analysis from the Framingham study showed that obesity and smoking each reduce life expectancy after the age 40 years, more so if combined together.

Competing interests: SHW has received a fee for speaking from Bayer. CDB has received honorariums and educational grants from several pharmaceutical companies involved in selling and developing treatments for obesity, cardiovascular disease, and diabetes.

> Clinical trials have shown the benefits of weight loss to improve dyslipidaemia, and exercise seems to have an additional benefit over the effects of a low fat diet. One review has reported that every kilogram of weight loss is associated with the following changes in lipid concentrations: fasting serum cholesterol −1.0%, LDL (low density lipoprotein) cholesterol −0.7%, triglycerides −1.9%, HDL cholesterol 0.2%

Lifestyle modification before drugs

- In 14 statin trials the mean LDL cholesterol concentration was 3.8 mmol/l and the average reduction in LDL cholesterol concentration was 1.1 mmol/l
- An average of over 40 kg of weight loss would be required to achieve an equivalent LDL reduction
- Clearly, to achieve cholesterol targets, many people require drug therapy as well as trying to lose weight. Weight loss alone can be very effective in improving lipid patterns in some overweight people
- Given the additional health benefits of weight loss and the potential side effects of drugs, lifestyle modification should always be tried first

Effects of obesity and smoking on life expectancy after age 40 on basis of follow-up data from Framingham study. Adapted from Peeters et al (see Further Reading box)

Study group*	Comparison group*	Years of life lost after age 40 relative to comparison group	
		Men	Women
≥ 30, non-smokers	18.5-24.9, non-smokers	5.8	7.1
≥ 30, smokers	BMI 18.5-24.9, smokers	6.7	7.2
≥ 30, smokers	BMI 18.5-24.9, non-smokers	13.7	13.3

*Body mass index and smoking status.

Further reading

- Colditz GA, Willett WC, Rotnitzky A, Manson JE. Weight gain as a risk factor for clinical diabetes mellitus in women. *Ann Intern Med* 1995;122:481-6.
- Must A, Spadano J, Coakley EH, Field AE, Colditz G, Dietz WH. The disease burden associated with overweight and obesity. *JAMA* 1999;282:1523-9.
- Byrne CD, Wild SH, eds. *The metabolic syndrome*. Chichester: Wiley, 2005.
- Peeters A, Barendregt JJ, Willekens F, Mackenbach JP, Al Mamun A, Bonneux L. Obesity in adulthood and its consequences for life expectancy: a life-table analysis. *Ann Intern Med* 2003;138:24-32.
- Norris SL, Zhang X, Avenell A, Gregg E, Brown TJ, Schmid CH, et al. Long-term non-pharmacologic weight loss interventions for adults with type 2 diabetes. *Cochrane Database Syst Rev* 2005;(2):CD004095.
- Sattar N, Tan CE, Han TS, Forster L, Lean ME, Shepherd J, et al. Associations of indices of adiposity with atherogenic lipoprotein subfractions. *Int J Obes Relat Metab Disord* 1998;22:432-9.

8   Obesity and vascular disease

Debbie A Lawlor, Mike Lean, Naveed Sattar

Previous articles in this series have discussed the relation of overweight and obesity with coronary heart disease (CHD) and individual cardiovascular disease risk factors—such as diabetes, raised blood pressure, and dyslipidaemia. This article examines the wider impact of obesity on vascular disease: the effect on cardiovascular disease of obesity as primary cause of the metabolic syndrome and of obesity as a risk factor for heart failure, stroke, other vascular conditions, and cognitive decline.

Metabolic syndrome

The metabolic syndrome refers to the clustering within individuals of several CHD risk factors—including glucose intolerance, dyslipidaemia, and raised blood pressure—believed to be linked by a common pathophysiological process. Individuals may develop these factors in different orders, with different severities, and at different ages, but they are unified by the fact that adult weight gain is a risk factor in their development. Reaven suggested in 1988 that insulin resistance was important in causing these risk factors, but others have concluded that obesity, particularly intra-abdominal fat accumulation, is probably a common primary cause.

Environmental exposures throughout life (such as high fat, energy dense diets; low levels of physical activity in childhood and adulthood; and factors related to poor intrauterine growth) also contribute to development of the metabolic syndrome. The (unknown) genetic predisposition is probably present in about 20-30% of all people.

Three definitions of the metabolic syndrome have been developed. A review in 2005 by Kahn et al (see Further Reading box) questions the clinical value of the syndrome.

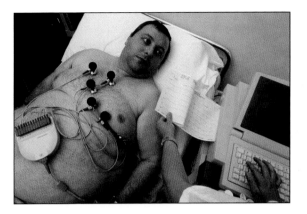

Definitions of insulin resistance

Broad definition

Insulin resistance is a clinical state in which a normal or raised insulin level produces an impaired biological response. As insulin has a number of physiological actions—including a central role in acute metabolic actions and growth and development—insulin resistance could mean impairment in any of these actions

Specific definition in relation to metabolic syndrome

Insulin resistance, when used to identify those at risk of type 2 diabetes and as a component of the metabolic syndrome, usually refers to resistance to insulin's ability to stimulate glucose uptake in insulin sensitive peripheral tissues and its ability to suppress hepatic glucose production, promote glucose storage, inhibit ketogenesis, and suppress lipolysis

Ethnic and sex specific definitions of obesity (based on waist circumference) used in the International Diabetes Federation's definition of metabolic syndrome

Ethnic group	Waist circumference (women; men)
Europids	≥ 80 cm; ≥ 94 cm
South Asians, Chinese, Japanese	≥ 80 cm; ≥ 90 cm
Ethnic south and central Americans	Use data for South Asians pending more specific research data
Sub-Saharan Africans; eastern Mediterranean and middle eastern (Arab) populations	Use data for Europids pending more specific research data

Summary definitions of metabolic syndrome

World Health Organization*
- Insulin resistance plus at least two of the following: raised blood pressure, dyslipidaemia, obesity, microalbuminuria

American Treatment Panel III†
At least three of the following:
- High fasting glucose
- Raised blood pressure
- Raised plasma triglycerides
- Low HDL (high density lipoprotein) cholesterol
- Obesity (large waist circumference)

International Diabetes Federation‡
- Obesity (large waist) plus at least two of the following: raised triglycerides, reduced HDL cholesterol, raised blood pressure, raised fasting plasma glucose

*Alberti K, Zimmet P. Definition, diagnosis and classification of diabetes mellitus and its complications. Part I: diagnosis and classification of diabetes mellitus provisional report of a WHO consultation. *Diabet Med* 1998;15:539-53.

†Executive Summary of the Third Report of the National Cholesterol Education Program (NCEP) Expert Panel on Detection, Evaluation, and Treatment of High Blood Cholesterol in Adults (Adult Treatment Panel III). *JAMA* 2001;285:2486-97.

‡International Diabetes Federation. *The IDF consensus worldwide definition of the metabolic syndrome.* 2005. www.idf.org/webdata/docs/Metac_syndrome_def.pdf (accessed 19 Sep 2006)

There are several problems with using a "diagnosis" of the metabolic syndrome (on the basis of the three definitions) as a screening test to identify people who would benefit from an intervention to improve cardiovascular health (such as weight management). The definitions use arbitrary thresholds for risk factors that are mostly linearly associated with cardiovascular disease. Despite the widespread practice of using thresholds of continuous risk factors to make "diagnoses" so that treatment can be started (for example, diagnosing hypertension on the basis of a blood pressure > 140/90 mm Hg), it is now technically possible to be more accurate in predicting disease risk.

The requirement for specific combinations of risk factors means that some individuals who are at risk of cardiovascular disease will not be diagnosed with the syndrome. The extent to which different risk factors matter will vary by sex, age, and ethnic group, and therefore the definitions will perform differently in different populations.

These issues are illustrated with an example from a study of British women aged 60-79 years. In this study there were similar weak associations of all three definitions of metabolic syndrome with incident CHD but greater association from hypertension. As hypertension is common in this age group, its absolute effect on CHD is high, whereas that of the metabolic syndrome (by any of the three definitions) is not. Obesity, however, was not an important predictor in this study.

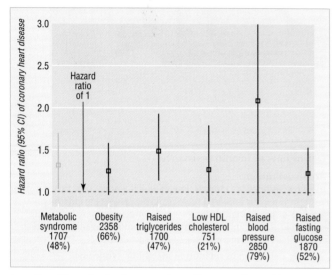
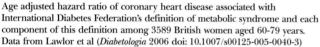

Age adjusted hazard ratio of coronary heart disease associated with International Diabetes Federation's definition of metabolic syndrome and each component of this definition among 3589 British women aged 60-79 years. Data from Lawlor et al (*Diabetologia* 2006 doi: 10.1007/s00125-005-0040-3)

Other studies have found that body mass index (weight in kilograms divided by height in metres squared) does not predict CHD in older individuals, probably reflecting a proportionately greater loss of lean muscle than fat with increased age. Thus, to reduce CHD in older women, assessing and appropriately treating raised blood pressure may be more important than diagnosing and treating the metabolic syndrome. Metabolic syndrome may, however, be a more potent predictor in younger subjects (say, <50 years) with premature CHD, as suggested by recent studies. This important point requires greater study, given the rising prevalence of obesity and its potentially greater impact on vascular risk in younger subjects.

For clinical practice we therefore need to develop more sophisticated risk prediction scores. Many primary care staff already have computer based, user friendly systems for estimating Framingham risk scores. An easy to use computer package could be developed that combines information on metabolic syndrome components and all other risk factors of an individual to give the best information about an individual's risk. In the meantime, to target obesity, a practical alternative strategy needs to recognise the importance of weight management in conjunction with cardiovascular disease risk.

Although obesity (in particular intra-abdominal fat accumulation), insulin resistance, diabetes risk, and cardiovascular disease risk are all associated with each other, models to predict cardiovascular disease are likely to differ from those used to predict type 2 diabetes. This is because some risk factors are specific to one but not the other. For example, raised

Potential weaknesses of current criteria for metabolic syndrome for predicting risk

- The current criteria have not yet been shown definitively to add to risk prediction for cardiovascular disease beyond current charts
- Arbitrary thresholds for risk factors and differing combinations of risk factors in the different definitions may lead to loss of important information about an individual's risk of cardiovascular disease
- The criteria fail to include important risk factors such as age, low density lipoprotein cholesterol, and smoking—a weakness if metabolic syndrome is used as the sole means of defining cardiovascular disease risk
- Prediction models that include additional risk factors (not just components of the metabolic syndrome) are a better means of identifying those at greatest risk

Requirements of future research

- Identify the best prediction models for cardiovascular disease and diabetes in different population groups (by pooling data from large number of individual prospective data sets in different populations)
- Evaluate the long term effect on disease risk of using these prediction models in clinical practice
- Determine the long term effect of weight maintenance and reduction programmes on cardiovascular disease risk using appropriately resourced and powered prospective trials

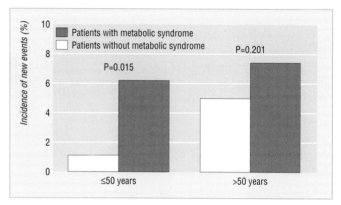

Age stratified incidence of new cardiovascular events (myocardial infarction, revascularisation, cardiac death) in patients with or without metabolic syndrome (according to modified criteria of American Treatment Panel III). Adapted from Reinhard et al (*Am J Cardiol* 2006;97:964-7)

Practical strategy for managing raised waist circumference in relation to cardiovascular disease risk

Waist /score for cardiovascular risk	Treatment
Circumference <80 cm in women, <94 cm in men (low risk)	Requires no intervention (avoid weight gain and stay below these levels)
Circumference ≥80 cm in women, ≥94 cm men, and <10% risk of cardiovascular disease* over next 10 years (raised risk)	Requires health promotion and public health measures for self directed treatment to prevent further weight gain
Circumference 80-88 cm in women and 94-102 cm men, and >10% risk of cardiovascular disease* over next 10 years (high risk)	Requires effective treatment to lose 5-10% body weight and to prevent further weight gain
Circumference >88 cm in women and >102 cm in men irrespective of 10 year risk of cardiovascular disease* (high risk for other medical problems associated with obesity or intra-abdominal fat accumulation)	Requires effective treatment to lose 5-10% body weight and to prevent further weight gain

*Risk based on Joint British Society's guidelines (or equivalent); cardiovascular risk score of >20% requires management in line with the society's guidelines

concentration of low density lipoprotein (LDL) cholesterol is a specific cardiovascular disease risk factor, and the metabolic syndrome is a stronger predictor of type 2 diabetes than it is of cardiovascular disease (see Sattar, Further Reading box.) However, studies using a variety of methods have found that people with metabolic syndrome (any definition) show a wide range of insulin sensitisation.

Potential bias and confounding

Three potential sources of bias could lead to underestimation of the effect of obesity on the development of vascular disease.

Firstly, as individuals developing cardiac disease may start to lose weight before the disease is diagnosed, reverse causality can explain null or weak findings. This can be avoided if only healthy individuals (at baseline) are included and long term prospective cohort studies are conducted.

Secondly, smoking is linked with lower body mass index (though larger waist), and so the underweight and "normal" weight categories (based on body mass index) will be over-represented with individuals who smoke. As smoking raises the risk of cardiovascular disease it can mask the effect of overweight and obesity on cardiovascular disease outcomes.

Thirdly, patients who are at high risk of cardiovascular disease (for example, those with a family history) may intentionally lose weight, and if this is not taken into account in the study design or analysis it again will result in an underestimation of the true effect of obesity on disease risk.

Heart failure

Overweight and obesity are associated with left ventricular hypertrophy and dilatation, which are known precursors of heart failure.

In the Framingham prospective cohort the incidence of heart failure gradually increased with greater body mass index, with the risk doubling in obese individuals. This increased risk was not fully explained by other risk factors, such as hypertension, raised cholesterol concentration, and diabetes, which had previously been thought to mediate the effect of obesity on heart failure. Obesity alone accounted for 11% of cases of heart failure in men and 14% of cases in women.

Similarly, results from the recently reported Uppsala longitudinal study of adult men found that greater body mass index and waist circumference were each associated with an increased risk of congestive heart failure in models that adjusted for diabetes, prior myocardial infarction, left ventricular hypertrophy, smoking, and serum cholesterol concentration. The study found strong evidence that insulin resistance might mediate the effect of obesity on heart failure.

Stroke

Several long term prospective cohort studies have found a strong association between greater body mass index or relative weight and risk of either total stroke or ischaemic stroke. The effect is attenuated by adjustment for risk factors such as hypertension, raised cholesterol concentration, and glucose intolerance. These risk factors are likely to be on the causal pathway between obesity and stroke, and therefore the attenuation of effect with their adjustment should not be interpreted as indicating that obesity is not causally related to stroke risk.

The effect of obesity on haemorrhagic stroke is less well established, but a large prospective cohort study of Korean men found a positive linear association between body mass index

Glucose, waist circumference, and triglyceride—three of the key components of the criteria for metabolic syndrome—are far stronger predictors of diabetes than of cardiovascular disease

The outlined conclusions on the associations of obesity with heart failure, stroke, and cognitive decline are based on the best available published evidence from prospective cohort studies that have used measures to minimise these sources of bias

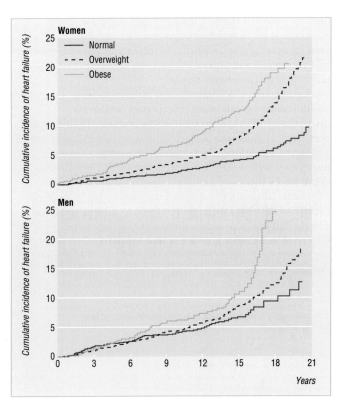

Cumulative incidence of heart failure by weight category (based on body mass index) at baseline examination in Framingham study. Adapted from Kenchaiah et al (see Further Reading box)

Survival in obese patients with heart failure

- An apparent survival advantage associated with higher body mass index in patients with heart failure does not mean that obesity is protective. Rather, a combination of earlier presentation of heart failure in obese subjects (due to symptoms at less severe levels of heart failure) and possibly reverse causality (non-purposeful weight loss in patients with heart failure who have a lower BMI associated with worse prognosis) may partly explain this "obesity paradox"
- Purposeful weight loss in heart failure patients with morbid obesity has been associated with improvements in systolic and diastolic function and in heart failure severity
- However, sufficiently powered randomised trials are needed to establish the effectiveness of weight reduction programmes in obese heart failure patients in relation to event-free survival

Obesity is also associated with increased risk of atrial fibrillation, venous thromboembolism, and sudden death. Obesity is therefore associated with a broad range of fatal and non-fatal cardiovascular events

and ischaemic stroke and a J shaped association with haemorrhagic stroke. Thus, for both ischaemic and haemorrhagic stroke, individuals with a body mass index above the reference category of 22-23 were at increased risk.

Cognitive decline

A recent prospective study of over 10 000 individuals whose weight, height, and subscapular and triceps skinfold thickness were assessed between 1964 and 1973 found that those who were overweight or obese (defined by body mass index) were at increased risk of dementia (that is, as recorded in their medical notes between 1994 and 2003).

The study also found positive linear associations between both measures of skinfold thickness and dementia. These associations remained after adjustment for potential confounders (age, sex, ethnicity, marital status, alcohol, smoking, and education) and potential mediating factors (hypertension, diabetes, high cholesterol, stroke).

As dementia was obtained from medical records, "confounding by indication" may in part explain the association: individuals who are obese are more likely to visit their doctors and more likely to be assessed for the presence of a range of conditions. Thus, it would be useful to see this association repeated in a prospective study that assessed dementia by means of a clinical interview with all cohort members. The authors suggested that obesity might increase the risk of dementia through its effect on diabetes and heart disease and may also have a direct effect on neuronal degradation. Emerging evidence also supports a link between higher physical activity levels and reduced risk of cognitive decline.

The photograph is published with permission from Mauro Fermariello/SPL.

Conclusion

- Clear evidence exists that obesity has a wider impact on cardiovascular health beyond its effect on coronary heart disease
- Individuals who are obese in mid-life are at increased risk of heart failure and stroke in later life, and emerging evidence shows that they may also be at increased risk of dementia. For all these associations, the link between obesity and disease outcome could result from the behaviours that cause adult weight gain—namely, inactivity and high fat diets
- Further, the associations may in part be mediated by obesity related diabetes, hypertension, and dyslipidaemia, but the causal pathway still involves adult weight gain. This emphasises the importance of reversing the current obesity epidemic, not only because of its impact on premature mortality but because of the devastating effect it will have on quality of life in older age through its impact on these disease outcomes

Further reading

- Kahn R, Buse J, Ferrannini E, Stern M. The metabolic syndrome: time for a critical appraisal: joint statement from the American Diabetes Association and the European Association for the Study of Diabetes. *Diabetes Care* 2005;28:2289-304.
- Sattar N. The metabolic syndrome: should current criteria influence clinical practice? *Curr Opin Lipidol* 2006;17:404-11.
- Kenchaiah S, Evans JC, Levy D, Wilson PW, Benjamin EJ, Larson MG, et al. Obesity and the risk of heart failure. *N Engl J Med* 2002;347:305-13.
- Ingelsson E, Sundstrom J, Arnlov J, Zethelius B, Lind L. Insulin resistance and risk of congestive heart failure. *JAMA* 2005;294:334-41.
- Lavie CJ, Mehra MR, Milani RV. Obesity and heart failure prognosis: paradox of reverse epidemiology? *Eur Heart J* 2005;26:5-7.
- Song Y-M, Sung J, Davey Smith G, Ebrahim S. Body mass index and ischemic and hemorrhagic stroke. A prospective study in Korean men. *Stroke* 2004;35:831-6.
- Murphy NF, MacIntyre K, Stewart S, Hart CL, Hole D, McMurray JJ. Long-term cardiovascular consequences of obesity: 20-year follow-up of more than 15 000 middle-aged men and women (the Renfrew-Paisley study). *Eur Heart J* 2006;27:96-106.
- Whitmer RA, Gunderson EP, Barrett-Connor E, Quesenberry CP Jr, Yaffe K. Obesity in middle age and future risk of dementia: a 27 year longitudinal population based study. *BMJ* 2005;330:1360-5.
- British Cardiac Society et al. Joint British societies' guidelines on prevention of cardiovascular disease in clinical practice. *Heart* 2005;91(suppl 5):v1-52.

9   Obesity and cancer

Donald C McMillan, Naveed Sattar, Mike Lean, Colin S McArdle

Incidence and mortality

Obesity is increasing at an alarming rate throughout North America and Europe and is associated with substantial morbidity and mortality. The condition has long been recognised as a risk factor for diabetes and cardiovascular disease, but not for developing cancer. A recent survey of the public by the American Cancer Society found that less than 5% of respondents were aware of the increased cancer risk associated with overweight and obesity.

A recent meta-analysis showed that more than 70 000 of the 3.5 million new cases of cancer each year in the European Union are attributable to overweight or obesity. This is likely to be a conservative estimate for two reasons. Firstly, only those tumours for which there was existing evidence to suggest a link between obesity and cancer (namely, for breast, colon, endometrium, prostate, kidney, and gallbladder) were included in the study. Secondly, the number of cancers attributable to obesity is likely to have increased because obesity levels have increased substantially since the publication of many of the studies included in this meta-analysis.

More recently, the American Cancer Society's prospective population based study of about 900 000 subjects confirmed that obesity was directly associated with an increased risk of death from a variety of cancers.

In both men and women, obesity was significantly associated with higher death rates from cancer of the oesophagus, colon and rectum, gallbladder, pancreas, and kidney, independently of smoking. Obesity was also associated with an increased risk of death from cancers of the stomach and prostate in men and from cancers of the breast (postmenopausal), uterus, cervix, and ovary in women. The increased risk of cancer has been most clearly defined in the common cancers. For example, in males the risk of colorectal cancer increased up to 80% in those whose body mass index (weight in kilograms divided by height in metres squared) was greater than 30.

Percentage of cancer cases attributable to overweight and obesity in countries of the European Union, by cancer site. Adapted from Bergstrom et al (see Further Reading box)

Site	Men	Women
Breast	*0*	*8.5*
Colon	11.1	10.7
Endometrium	NA	39.2
Prostate	4.4	NA
Kidney	25.5	24.5
Gall bladder	24.8	23.7
All cancers	3.4	6.4

NA = not applicable.

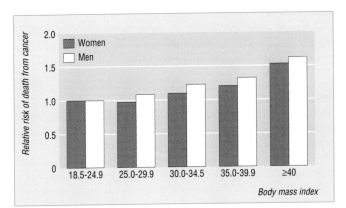

Contribution of overweight and obesity to mortality from cancer in the United States, 1982-98. Adapted from Adami H-O et al (*N Engl J Med* 2003;348:1623-4)

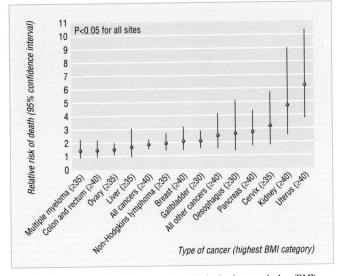

Mortality from cancer for US women, 1982-98, by body mass index (BMI). For each relative risk, the comparison was between women in the highest BMI category and women in the reference category (18.5 to 24.9). Adapted from Calle et al (see Further Reading box)

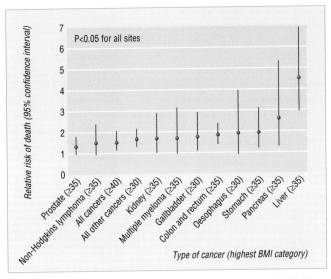

Mortality from cancer for US men, 1982-98, by body mass index (BMI). For each relative risk, the comparison was between men in the highest BMI category and men in the reference category (18.5 to 24.9). Adapted from Calle et al (see Further Reading box)

On the basis of these results from the American Cancer Society, overweight and obesity in the United States is currently estimated to account for 14% of all deaths from cancer in men and 20% of those in women. Taken together, this means that 90 000 cancer deaths could be prevented each year if Americans could maintain a healthy body weight. In Europe, 9000 of the 70 000 cancer cases attributable to obesity and overweight ("avoidable" cases) are in the United Kingdom.

Role of lifestyle factors

Diet
Many studies have tried to document the health hazard that can be related to a diet high in calories and animal fat and low in fibre, fruit, and vegetables—a diet typical of Western market economies. Surveys of eating habits are consistently confounded by under-reporting, particularly among obese respondents.

Although initial studies suggested a strong association with total fat intake, particularly from animal sources, recent findings from retrospective and prospective epidemiological studies have been inconsistent. In addition, cereals with high fibre content have been associated with a lower risk of colorectal cancer, yet several large population based studies have failed to show benefit.

A more consistent association exists between reduced risk of cancer and increased consumption of a wide variety of fruit and vegetables; however, the relative quantities of each required to reduce risk is not known.

Physical activity
On the basis of existing evidence, public health organisations have issued guidelines for preventing chronic diseases including cancer. These recommendations include more exercise during daily routine—for example, use stairs, walk to work, walk in the park, and do more physical activity around the home (such as gardening). Specifically, individuals are advised to do some sustained physical activity—such as brisk walking for 30-40 minutes—at least five days a week. For people with known cardiovascular disease, a lower level of physical activity may be of benefit— however, they should do this only after consultation with their doctor.

A recent population based study of adults in 48 states in North America has shown an increase in obesity in all states and a decrease in physical activity in only 11. This suggests that obesity is now primarily diet induced, the result of a sustained excess of energy rich foods with high fat and refined carbohydrate content, as well as an insufficient consumption of fruit and vegetables. This is compounded by increasingly sedentary lifestyles; paradoxically, appetite is increased in inactive people.

In Europe, the position is less clear as some evidence exists to suggest that the lack of physical activity may make a more important contribution to the development of obesity.

Mechanisms

Several plausible biological mechanisms have been suggested to explain the relation between obesity and the increased risk of developing cancer, including the increased concentrations of endogenous hormones. These hormones (sex steroids, insulin, and insulin growth factor-1) are increased with the accumulation of body fat and are important in the control of growth, differentiation, and metabolism of cells. In particular, hyperinsulinaemia would link obesity related cancer with the high energy, highly processed, carbohydrate and animal fat diet

> Given that obesity rates in European countries are fast catching up with those in North America, similar numbers of patients will probably be exposed to an increased risk of developing cancer

> The relation between obesity and the incidence of cancers is likely to be linked to aspects of lifestyle—in particular, diet and physical activity

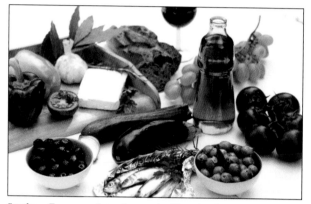

Southern European diets—characterised by a low intake of animal fat and a high intake of fish, olive oil, vegetables, fruits, and grain—are consistently associated with lower rates of cancer

> Almost 170 observational studies have evaluated the relation between physical activity and the risk of developing cancer. The results of these studies provide convincing evidence that increased physical activity is associated with a reduction in several common solid tumours, including colon cancer

The balance between energy intake and expenditure
- In some people the major issue is overeating for the physical activity they perform
- In others, the major issue is too little physical activity and a failure to reduce their food intake accordingly
- Therefore, in both cases, obesity seems to result from an inability to match energy intake and energy expenditure

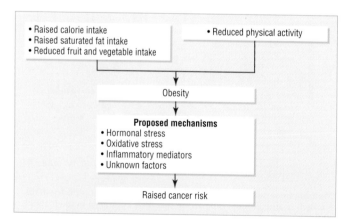

Links between obesity, lifestyle factors, and risk for cancer

typical of Western society. It is therefore of interest that patients with type 2 diabetes are known to have increased rates of cancer.

Chronic inflammation is recognised to be an important factor in the initiation and promotion of cancer cells. Recent studies suggest that adipocytes are a potent source of pro-inflammatory cytokines and that obesity is a key component explaining the presence of a chronic, low grade, systemic inflammatory response in the general population.

The presence of a systemic inflammatory response (as evidenced by an increase in circulating C reactive protein concentrations) has been shown, for example, to be associated with an increased risk of colorectal cancer. These observations are consistent with the results of recent randomised trials showing that the use of conventional non-steroidal anti-inflammatory drugs reduce the incidence of polyp formation. Therefore, the presence of a chronic systemic inflammatory response provides a potential direct link between obesity and increased development of cancer. Obesity is linked to enhanced oxidative stress, in part through the inflammatory process, and increased oxidative damage to DNA could raise cancer risk.

Guidelines

Sufficient evidence exists that the incidence of cancer can be reduced by changes in lifestyle to include a healthy diet and physical activity. The International Union Against Cancer (UICC) has issued dietary guidelines for reducing cancer risk.

Conclusion

Obesity in the United Kingdom is increasing rapidly and will lead to an increase not only in the incidence of diabetes and cardiovascular disease but also in the incidence of cancer. It remains to be seen whether a documented excess risk of death due to cancer among overweight and obese people will provide additional motivation for controlling body weight around the world.

The photograph is published with permission from Alix/Phanie/Rex.

Guidelines of the International Union Against Cancer

Consume a lifelong, varied diet rich in plant foods
- Include fruits and vegetables in every meal
- Eat fruits and vegetables as snacks
- Substitute beans for meat
- Select wholegrain products rather than refined grains
- Include high fibre foods in the diet

Restrict intake of fatty foods
- Meat portions should be small relative to servings of plant food
- Meat should be trimmed of fat
- Eat fish and poultry rather than meats high in saturated fats
- Limit intake of fried food
- Limit additions of fats and oils to prepared foods
- Limit or avoid alcohol consumption

Store and prepare foods in ways that reduce contamination
- Fresh foods should be properly cleaned before consumption
- Perishable foods should be refrigerated
- Limit consumption of salted, nitrite treated, smoked, and pickled foods
- Avoid charred foods, which can be carcinogenic
- Add less salt during food preparation and eating

Balance dietary intake and energy expenditure to avoid excesses of high or low weight
- Eat small portions of high energy foods
- Exercise to maintain weight

Do not rely on supplementary vitamins and minerals as substitutes for balanced and adequate diet
- Maximise intake of essential nutrients by inclusion of vitamin and mineral rich foods
- Use supplements only for needs not adequately met by diet

Further reading and resources
- Bergstrom A, Pisani P, Tenet V, Wolk A, Adami HO. Overweight as an avoidable cause of cancer in Europe. *Int J Cancer* 2001;91:421-30.
- Calle EE, Rodriguez C, Walker-Thurmond K, Thun MJ. Overweight, obesity, and mortality from cancer in a prospectively studied cohort of US adults. *N Engl J Med* 2003;348:1625-38.
- Vigneri P, Frasca F, Sciacca L, Frittitta L, Vigneri R. Obesity and cancer. *Nutr Metab Cardiovasc Dis* 2006;16:1-7.
- www.iotf.org (International Association for the Study of Obesity)
- www.uicc.org (International Union Against Cancer)
- www.wcrf.org (World Cancer Research Fund)
- www.iarc.fr (International Agency for Research on Cancer)

10 Obesity and reproduction

Jane E Ramsay, Ian Greer, Naveed Sattar

The effect of adiposity is manifest in nearly every aspect of female reproductive life, whether as a metabolic or reproductive complication or as a technical problem affecting clinical issues such as ultrasonography or surgery. Indeed, obesity is present in 35% of maternal deaths in the United Kingdom.

Such concerns are particularly important given recent evidence of a doubling in the prevalence of obesity in young women attending for antenatal care in maternity hospitals in the UK (in some places, almost one in five are now obese). In the United States, where obesity rates are generally even higher, the American College of Obstetricians and Gynecologists has issued guidance on the impact of obesity on pregnancy.

Gynaecological concerns

Strong evidence shows that insulin resistance is an integral part of polycystic ovarian syndrome, especially in obese women. In most women with the syndrome, hyperinsulinaemia—driven or revealed by excess weight gain—promotes ovarian androgen secretion and abnormal follicular development, leading to dysfunctional ovarian and menstrual activity.

Androgens are carried in the circulation bound to sex hormone binding globulin (SHBG). Conditions of high androgen and insulin concentrations are associated with lower levels of SHBG, resulting in high free androgen activity. Thus, clinical manifestations of polycystic ovarian syndrome are associated with androgen activity and include hirsutism, acne, and alopecia, as well as oligomenorrhoea and ovulation failure.

Medications that contain oestrogen (such as the combined contraceptive pill) or ovulation induction drugs (resulting in high levels of endogenous oestrogen) may be associated with an increased risk of venous thromboembolism in obese women. The combined effect of obesity and the combined contraceptive pill results in a 10-fold increased risk of venous thromboembolism in women with a body mass index of >25 (body mass index is calculated by dividing weight in kilograms by height in metres squared). Therefore routine management options for the gynaecological associations of obesity are to a certain extent contraindicated.

The potential for a significantly complicated pregnancy in obese women is high and therefore in a woman with impaired fertility owing to obesity, the ethical concern is whether to start medical management before a serious attempt at weight loss through diet and exercise.

Obstetric concerns

Subfertility treatment and early pregnancy outcome

Some data suggest that the most clinically useful predictors of poor outcome from gonadotrophin ovulation induction in women with normogonadotrophic anovulatory infertility are obesity and insulin resistance. Also, an obese woman is three times more likely to miscarry. This association further emphasises the importance of encouraging weight loss to maximise the chance of a successful pregnancy before starting to treat anovulatory subfertility.

Potential effects of adiposity before and during pregnancy

	Medical complications	Technical complications
Prepregnancy	Menstrual disorders, infertility	
Early pregnancy	Miscarriage, fetal anomalies	Difficult ultrasound examination
Antenatal	Pregnancy induced hypertension, pre-eclampsia, gestational diabetes, venous thromboembolism	
Intrapartum	Induction of labour, shoulder dystocia, caesarean section	Operative or anaesthetic problems
Postpartum	Haemorrhage, infection, venous thromboembolism	
Fetal	Macrosomia, fetal distress, perinatal morbidity/mortality	Birth injury

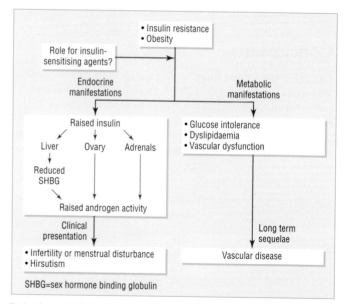

Endocrine and clinical effects of obesity and insulin resistance in women. Adapted from Harborne et al. *Lancet* 2003;361:1894-901

Obese women are about three times as likely as non-obese women to have an infant with either spina bifida or an omphalocele and about twice as likely to have a baby with either a heart defect or multiple anomalies

Although folic acid supplementation before conception is recommended for all women, the increased risk of neural tube defects in obese women has persisted in populations where flour has been fortified with folic acid

Risks of pregnancy complications associated with obesity, according to five studies. Risks expressed as odds ratio (95% confidence interval) or percentage (US cohort study)

Study (by complication)	Risk of complication
Miscarriage	
Meta-analysis (13 studies) in women with normogonadotrophic anovulatory infertility examined patient predictors for outcome of ovulation induction with gonadotrophins: obese *v* non-obese women	Rate of spontaneous miscarriage (3.05 (1.4 to 6.4))
Fetal anomalies	
Case-control study of major birth defects in about 40 000 births/year in 1993-97	Spina bifida 3.5 (1.2 to 10.3), omphalocele 3.3 (1.0 to 10.3), heart defects 2.0 (1.2 to 3.4)
All complications	
UK study of 287 213 singleton pregnancies (62% normal weight, 28% overweight, 11% obese): obese versus normal weight	Gestational diabetes 3.6 (3.25 to 3.98), pre-eclamptic toxaemia 2.14 (1.85 to 2.47), macrosomia 2.36 (2.23 to 2.50), intrauterine death 1.4 (1.14 to 1.71), induction of labour 1.70 (1.64 to 1.76), caesarean section 1.83 (1.74 to 1.93), postpartum haemorrhage 1.39 (1.32 to 1.46), genital infection 1.3 (1.1 to 1.6), urinary tract infection 1.4 (1.2 to 1.6), wound infection 2.2 (2.0 to 2.6)
US cohort study of 613 morbidly obese and 11 313 non-obese women	Gestational diabetes 14% *v* 4%, pre-eclamptic toxaemia 14% *v* 3.2%, fetal distress 12% *v* 8%, caesarean section 31% *v* 15%, endometritis 9% *v* 3%
Case control study from Middle East of 159 obese women and 300 women of normal weight, matched for age and parity	Gestational diabetes mellitus 26 (9 to 73), pregnancy induced hypertension 11 (5 to 24), caesarean section 1.9 (1.1 to 3.4), macrosomia 3.3 (2.0 to 5.5)

Metabolic complications

Hypertension

The risks of pregnancy induced hypertension or pre-eclampsia are significantly greater if the woman is overweight. Most published work suggests a twofold to threefold increase in risk of pre-eclampsia if early pregnancy body mass index (>30) or waist circumference (>88 cm) is used as an indicator of obesity.

Diabetes

Maternal obesity is associated with a fourfold increase in risk of gestational diabetes. In the short term, appropriate management of gestational diabetes can reduce the incidence of fetal macrosomia and serious perinatal morbidity, although it can increase the need for intervention.

In the long term, women with gestational diabetes are much more likely (severalfold higher risk) than the general population to develop diabetes, and this risk may be greatest in obese women. Therefore, in obese women with gestational diabetes, the early postnatal visit is an ideal opportunity for lifestyle advice on weight loss and exercise. Such women should be regularly screened for type 2 diabetes.

Venous thromboembolism

Venous thromboembolism is the leading cause of maternal death in the UK. Pregnancy is a prothrombotic state, with increases in coagulation factors and a decrease in natural anticoagulants along with inhibition of fibrinolysis.

Other factors likely to be important in the aetiology of venous thromboembolism associated with pregnancy are obesity, advanced maternal age, high parity, operative delivery, and pre-eclampsia, with these last four also being associated with maternal obesity.

Technical concerns

Ultrasonography in morbidly obese patients can be challenging. Adipose tissue attenuates the ultrasound signal by absorption of the associated energy. Therefore a high frequency, higher resolution signal would be more significantly absorbed at a lesser depth, requiring sacrifice of image quality for depth of field.

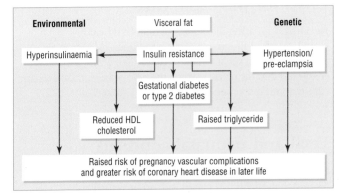

Adiposity, insulin resistance, and clinical effects in non-pregnant and pregnant women. A central body fat distribution can be influenced by both genetic and environmental factors. However, this phenotype is believed to be inextricably linked with the "metabolic syndrome." These factors are reflected in pre-eclampsia and gestational diabetes

> **Obesity seems to treble the risk of thrombosis, with greater likelihood of progression to pulmonary embolism, and obese individuals have higher levels of factor VIII and factor IX, but not of fibrinogen**

Potential technical problems in managing obese mothers

- Difficult to use ultrasonography accurately to date pregnancy or detect fetal anomalies
- Large cuffs required to measure blood pressure accurately
- Woman may have reduced awareness of fetal movements
- External electronic fetal monitoring can be problematical
- Surgery is technically difficult, requiring more assistants or larger operating table
- Regional and general anaesthesia can be challenging
- Wound care can be compromised in the event of caesarean section

A study of routine ultrasound screening in pregnant women with diabetes found that major congenital anomalies were almost six times as common in these women as in controls. The detection rate was significantly lower, however, for the diabetic women than for the controls (30% v 73%; P < 0.01), and this was related to the higher incidence of obesity. This is important, as even in obese women without diabetes, epidemiological evidence consistently shows an increased rate of fetal anomalies.

Increased rates of intrapartum complications (such as failure to progress, shoulder dystocia, induction of labour, and emergency caesarean section) occur in many different populations of obese women. With the increased rate of caesarean sections in obese women, anaesthesia services need to be effective.

Many emergency sections for cephalopelvic disproportion or failure to progress occur at night-time, when many labour wards are staffed by the most junior staff, both obstetric and anaesthetic. So the least experienced staff may perform the most technically demanding and consequently high risk surgery and anaesthesia. In women who have had a previous section, the chance of successful vaginal delivery is < 15% for those who are very obese.

Costs for maternal care

As obesity can affect all aspects of maternal health, management of pregnancy in obese women is likely to be associated with a substantial increase in cost. One study has suggested that for obese women the cost of hospital antenatal care is about five times higher than the average.

Fetal and neonatal concerns

Short term
Maternal obesity is associated with an increased risk of fetal macrosomia, and data show that the incidence of birth weight of ≥ 4000 g is increased, regardless of whether the mother has diabetes. Macrosomia is a risk factor for a lower Apgar score at 1 minute and a lower umbilical arterial pH level, as well as for severe injuries to the baby (fractures and palsies). The overall morbidity for these babies is increased by about 8%.

Data on risk of intrauterine growth restriction is conflicting. In general, intrauterine growth restriction does not seem to be associated with maternal obesity, which seems to protect against spontaneous preterm labour.

Despite this, the percentage of infants requiring admission to a neonatal intensive care unit seems to be significantly higher in children born to obese mothers, presumably secondary to the increased rates of antenatal complications and complications secondary to macrosomia. Obese women are also less likely to breast feed.

Long term
Research has suggested that impaired adult cardiovascular health may be programmed in utero by poor fetal nutrition, or by genetically determined attenuation of insulin mediated fetal growth, resulting in a small infant. Recent studies suggest, however, that obese mothers (even if they do not develop diabetes) may adversely programme their offspring in utero for greater obesity in later life (see Catalono, Further Reading box).

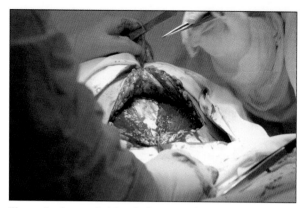

The mechanisms underlying the increased risks of intrapartum complications for obese women are elusive and do not simply reflect macrosomia. One hypothesis suggests increased soft tissue obstruction of labour, and dysfunctional uterine contractions may also be involved. In the postpartum period there is an increased rate of haemorrhage, genital tract infection, urinary tract infection, and wound infection

Why obesity can raise management costs of pregnancy

- Increased risk of admission to hospital for complications such as pre-eclampsia
- Increased use of ultrasonography and operator time for difficult anomaly scans and fetal assessment
- Increased risk of operative delivery and postpartum complications such as infection, haemorrhage, and venous thromboembolism
- Increased risk of neonatal admission

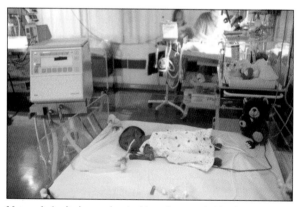

Maternal obesity is associated with an increased risk of neonates being admitted to a neonatal intensive care unit

Population based research shows a link between maternal obesity and cardiovascular disease in adult offspring. Also, higher adult rates of type 2 diabetes have been reported in offspring of mothers who were above average weight in pregnancy

Given that obesity and maternal insulin resistance is not only genetic but acquired, improvement of periconceptional maternal insulin sensitivity via activity or diet may affect not only a mother's health but also the future cardiovascular risk of her child. This hypothesis is speculative, however; further research is needed

Reproductive concerns in men

The prevalence of some degree of erectile dysfunction in men aged 40-70 years is thought to be about 50%. Symptoms are increased in obese men, and the underlying pathophysiology is believed to be associated with the complications of the metabolic syndrome. In the past decade, erectile dysfunction has become a "hot topic" for developments in medical therapy. However, modifiable health behaviours, including weight loss and physical activity, are clearly associated with a reduced risk for erectile dysfunction.

Intervention and outcome

In obese women, we must consider modification of risk factors before, or early in, a pregnancy. Increased physical activity in women who are sedentary may result in a better pregnancy outcome for both mother and child. Preliminary data support this hypothesis, and some data also suggest beneficial effects of exercise in pregnancy on fetal development, showing significantly higher birth weights and faster mid-trimester growth rates. Larger trials are needed.

Exercise in pregnancy may also reduce pregnancy complications such as gestational diabetes and does not seem to be harmful, with no association with premature labour or poor Apgar scores. Data from the recent Cochrane meta-analysis on use of aspirin for prophylaxis of pre-eclampsia has suggested an overall reduction of risk of 15%. However, when aspirin is targeted at women in high risk groups—for example, when multiple risk factors exist (such as obesity, age, family history)—it may have a more significant effect.

Finally, because of the considerable potential adverse impact of obesity on pregnancy outcome for both mother and baby, some researchers have even suggested that surgical treatment of obesity in young women may be warranted to prevent such complications.

Advice for achieving a healthy lifestyle should be actively disseminated by all health professionals at every opportunity, including the gynaecology clinic and antenatal and postnatal visits. Ideally, the risks of conceiving when obese should be disseminated through public health initiatives. Prepregnancy clinics could provide education on healthy diet and exercise regimens that could be followed before trying to conceive.

The photographs of a caesarean section and a neonatal intensive care unit are published with permission from Jacky Chapman/Photofusion and Garry Watson/SPL respectively.

Suggestions for clinically managing pregnancy in obese women*

- Obese women should receive prepregnancy counselling (via clinics for subfertility, recurrent miscarriage, or diabetes; via obstetric prepregnancy clinics; or via a general practitioner) and folic acid supplements
- Encourage obese women to lose weight before conceiving, and to use contraception while aiming for target weight (fertility rises as body mass index decreases)
- Advise on the importance of healthy diet and exercise and the need to avoid excessive weight gain (refer to dietitian if necessary)
- Consider low dose aspirin in the presence of additional risk factors (obesity is associated with increased risk of pre-eclampsia); assess thrombosis risk and provide thromboprophylaxis if needed
- Recommend detailed anomaly scan and serum screening for congenital abnormality
- Consider glucose tolerance testing at 28 weeks
- Recommend anaesthetic review before delivery
- Plan delivery to allow optimum management by experienced obstetricians
- Consider prophylactic postpartum antibiotics if delivery is complicated
- Assess thrombosis risk postpartum and provide thromboprophylaxis if indicated
- Consider extended thromboprophylaxis after discharge
- Arrange postnatal review at six weeks to discuss any problems and potential for future intervention

*Best targeted at women with body mass index of >35 (rather than >30). Further data is needed for cost effectiveness of targeting all women with BMI >30 as this would have major impact on clinical practice owing to high prevalence (near 20%) of obesity in young women in some places, and thus needs a better evidence base

Further reading and resources

- Ramsay JE, Greer IA. Obesity in pregnancy. *Fetal Matern Med Rev* 2004;15:109-32.
- Kanagalingam MG, Forouhi NG, Greer IA, Sattar N. Changes in booking body mass index over a decade: retrospective analysis from a Glasgow maternity hospital. *BJOG* 2005;112:1431-3.
- Wong SF, Chan FY, Cincotta RB, Oats JJ, McIntyre HD. Routine ultrasound screening in diabetic pregnancies. *Ultrasound Obstet Gynecol* 2002;19:171-6.
- Galtier-Dereure F, Boegner C, Bringer J. Obesity and pregnancy: complications and cost. *Am J Clin Nutr* 2000;71:1242-8S.
- Callaway LK, Prins JB, Chang AM, McIntyre HD. The prevalence and impact of overweight and obesity in an Australian obstetric population. *Med J Aust* 2006;184:56-9.
- Catalano PM. Obesity and pregnancy—the propagation of a viscous cycle? *J Clin Endocrinol Metab* 2003;88:3505-6.
- American College of Obstetricians and Gynecologists' guidance on the impact of obesity on pregnancy. 2005. www.acog.org/from_home/publications/press_releases/nr08-31-05-2.cfm.

11 Childhood obesity

John J Reilly, David Wilson

Obesity, an excessive body fat content with increased risk of morbidity, has become increasingly common in children and adolescents. Confusion exists, however, over basic questions such as whether paediatric obesity matters, how to diagnose it, and whether it should be treated (and if so, how best to do this). Doctors in many fields need a better understanding of these issues.

Diagnosis

Subjective assessment methods are inaccurate, so diagnosis must be objective. A substantial and consistent body of high quality evidence has shown that body mass index (BMI; weight in kilograms divided by height in metres squared) can be used to diagnose obesity effectively.

BMI is lower in childhood and adolescence than in adulthood and differs between boys and girls. Clinically, no diagnostic alternative exists, therefore, to considering BMI in an age and sex specific manner, either by plotting it on a BMI chart or by referring to tables of BMI for age and sex.

In the United Kingdom, BMI for age charts represent the distribution of BMI in children in 1990. Diagnosing obesity as a high BMI centile (such as the 98th centile or above on the UK charts) identifies the fattest children in the population with high specificity (low false positive rate). High specificity provides confidence that a child diagnosed as obese in this way actually is excessively fat, and not simply muscular. In addition, strong evidence shows that children with a high BMI centile are at high risk of comorbid conditions, so the diagnosis is clinically meaningful.

For comparisons of obesity prevalence between nations, "international" definitions of overweight and obesity based on BMI for age are available. These are designed to provide definitions that are conceptually equivalent to adult BMI values of 25 and 30 respectively.

Despite high specificity for excess fatness, a high BMI for age has only modest sensitivity in children and adolescents (moderate false negative rate). Modest sensitivity is a problem for public health applications such as surveillance of obesity, as estimates of prevalence of obesity based on BMI tend to be conservative.

Future research may provide useful diagnostic alternatives to BMI, and the use of waist circumference in the paediatric age range is promising, though not yet sufficiently evidence based.

Prevalence

In the UK the epidemic of paediatric obesity began in the late 1980s. Prevalence has continued to increase rapidly, and obesity is now the most common disorder of childhood and adolescence. The health survey for England 2004 showed that 14% of 2-11 year olds and 25% of 11-15 year olds were obese (BMI ≥95th centile).

In the United States, prevalence of childhood obesity is highest in some ethnic minority groups; preliminary evidence suggests that this might also be the case in Europe, although further research is necessary and will require oversampling of children and adolescents from ethnic minority groups.

> **This chapter summarises recent evidence based clinical guidelines and systematic reviews and proposes strategies for managing paediatric obesity**

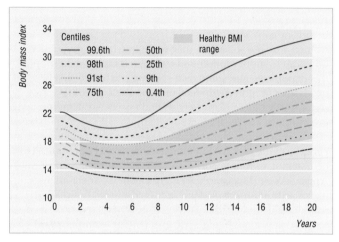

Simplified diagram of some body mass index curves seen on UK BMI charts for boys (that for girls is similar). The charts are available from Harlow Health via the Child Growth Foundation (www.childgrowthfoundation.org)

Evidence based definitions of paediatric obesity

For research and epidemiological purposes
- Overweight should be defined as BMI ≥85th centile for sex and age
- Obesity should be defined as BMI ≥95th centile for sex and age

For clinical purposes in UK
- Overweight should be defined as BMI ≥91st centile if using the UK BMI charts
- Obesity should be defined as BMI ≥98th centile if using the UK BMI charts

---

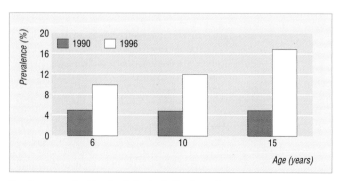

Development of epidemic of obesity in English children during the 1990s. Adapted from Reilly et al (Lancet 1999;354:1874-5)

Excess obesity is a particularly important clinical issue in certain ethnic groups, such as South Asians. South Asians are more sensitive to the adverse effects of excess weight gain and account for most childhood cases of type 2 diabetes in the UK.

Consequences of childhood obesity

A systematic review and critical appraisal recently concluded that paediatric obesity was a major health burden not only in childhood and adolescence but also later on, in adulthood.

Short term

Many obese patients seeking medical care experience teasing and bullying and will have low self esteem or a poor quality of life. Paediatric obesity is also associated with many other comorbid conditions. Evidence on some important comorbidities (such as liver disease) and on the adverse economic effects of paediatric obesity has only emerged recently, and the list of adverse consequences will lengthen in the near future.

From a public health viewpoint the most serious consequence of obesity in childhood may be its damaging long term effects on individuals' cardiovascular health. Cardiovascular risk factors are common, particularly in obese adolescents, and tend to "cluster" (aggregate) in obese individuals. For example, in a non-clinical sample of adolescents in the United States, 29% of those who were obese had the metabolic syndrome compared with 0.1% of those who were not overweight.

Long term

Evidence linking childhood obesity to adult disease and premature mortality is difficult to obtain and is currently limited. However, systematic review and critical appraisal is supportive of the hypothesis that paediatric obesity has adverse effects on health in adulthood.

Obesity tends to persist, particularly from adolescence into adulthood. Children are least likely to "grow out of" obesity when it is more severe and when they have at least one obese parent, and both of these features are much more common now than in the past. These days, at least 60% of obese children and 70-80% of obese adolescents are likely to become obese adults.

Prevention

The evidence on interventions for prevention has recently been reviewed systematically and critically appraised. Few randomised controlled trials have been conducted. Most trials were found to be methodologically weak and short term, and most of the interventions tested were unlikely to be generalisable.

Few trials found benefits linked to the intervention being tested. One notable exception, however, is the "Planet Health" intervention in US schoolchildren, which was of high methodological quality, reasonably long term, generalisable, and successful (at least in girls). The success of this particular intervention was attributed largely to reductions in television viewing.

Further research on preventive interventions is needed urgently. A helpful guide to preventive interventions was proposed by Whitaker. One barrier to such interventions is the common perception among parents, teachers, and health professionals that the interventions may cause harm (for example, by promoting eating disorders). Such adverse effects are extremely unlikely.

Obesity is more common in older children and adolescents than in younger children; in the developed world it is slightly more common in children from less affluent families, for reasons that are unclear

---

Consequences of paediatric obesity

Short term (for the child or adolescent)
- Psychological ill health
- Cardiovascular risk factors
- Asthma
- Chronic inflammation
- Diabetes (type 1 and 2)
- Orthopaedic abnormalities
- Liver disease

Long term (for the adult who was obese as a child or adolescent)
- Persistence of obesity
- Adverse socioeconomic outcomes, particularly in women
- Cardiovascular risk factors, diabetes, cancers, depression, arthritis
- Premature mortality

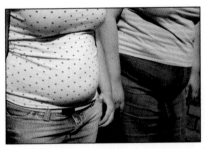

Obesity in adolescence, particularly in girls, is associated with impaired adult socioeconomic outcomes such as poorer educational results and lower income

---

"Planet Health" trial*

Intervention
- Was conducted over two school years; 1295 participants aged 11 years at baseline
- Aimed to reduce television viewing, increase lifestyle physical activity, reduce fat intake, and increase fruit and vegetable intake
- Intervention was tested rigorously in a high quality randomised trial
- Intervention is probably generalisable
- Assessment of economic impact was carried out

Outcomes
- School based changes were sustainable and cost effective
- Benefits to intervention were found in girls (reduced risk of becoming obese, remission of existing obesity)
- Benefits were attributed to reductions in television viewing

*Trial of model programme for school based obesity prevention (further details from Gortmaker et al. *Arch Pediatr Adolesc Med* 1999;151:409-15)

Guide to prevention interventions*

Interventions should:
- Do no harm
- Lead to benefiting child health or development in other ways
- Target behaviours that are causally related to the development of obesity or to its maintenance
- Target behaviours that are modifiable
- Target behaviours that are measurable because (a) families would otherwise find it difficult to make changes and (b) scientific evaluation requires measurement

*Modified and expanded from Whitaker (*Arch Pediatr Adolesc Med* 2003;157:725-7)

Treatment

Recent systematic reviews and critical appraisal exercises have consistently concluded that the evidence on interventions to treat paediatric obesity is extremely limited. Most of the randomised controlled trials have been methodologically weak and short term, and many have been unsuccessful. Most trials tested interventions that are unlikely to be generalisable. Systematic reviews have identified promising elements of treatment from the literature.

No high quality evidence is currently available on the medium to long term effects of surgical treatment, drug treatment, or residential treatment. Longer term randomised controlled trials of these forms of treatment are needed urgently.

Audits of typical dietetic and paediatric treatment of obesity in the US and in the UK usually report disappointing results. A recently conducted five year audit of an obesity clinic at the Royal Hospital for Sick Children in Edinburgh found that over half of the patients who had been referred to the clinic did not attend any of their appointments. Of the patients who attended at least one appointment, only 22% maintained their weight over six months.

Management

To know how to manage childhood obesity we need to know who should be treated, who should be referred, and what the treatment should aim for.

Systematic reviews and critical appraisals have concluded that the evidence base (from reports from expert committees) for providing answers to these questions is weak. Nevertheless, these reports are likely to be extremely helpful in management.

Summary of reports from expert committees

Who should be treated?

As treatment of obesity requires long term adherence to lifestyle changes, success is unlikely if patients and/or their family do not perceive obesity as a problem or if they are poorly motivated to make lifestyle changes.

The disappointing results of treatment from past audits partly reflect a lack of understanding among families that paediatric obesity matters. Treatment should be reserved for families who perceive obesity as a problem and who show motivation to make and sustain lifestyle changes.

Who should be referred?

Referral from primary to secondary care would be justified for two reasons: to investigate possible underlying pathological causes of the patient's obesity; and to investigate or manage a possible comorbid condition such as type 2 diabetes.

In the vast majority of patients obesity is caused by lifestyle; pathological causes are extremely rare. An underlying pathological cause should be suspected, however, if obesity is particularly severe in young children (where it may reflect an underlying genetic cause such as a single gene defect) or if it coexists with short stature (which may indicate a syndromic cause such as the Prader-Willi syndrome or some other endocrine cause).

If referral to secondary care reveals no comorbidities requiring urgent treatment and no underlying pathological causes of obesity, patients could be discharged to primary care for treatment. However, in many parts of the UK treatment of childhood obesity is either limited or not offered at all in primary or secondary care.

Useful tips when treating paediatric obesity

- Treat as "intensively" as possible—more frequent and longer appointments are beneficial
- Treat the whole family, not just the child
- Treat only motivated families
- Aim for dietary changes, perhaps using a "traffic light" approach—that is, greatly restrict foods high in energy ("red"); restrict foods with moderate energy content ("amber") to meal times only; eat freely foods that are low in energy ("green") and substitute them for red foods

---

The possibility of causing harm is also perceived by parents, teachers, and health professionals as a barrier to treatment, but the evidence suggests that this is unlikely. In fact, with some treatment interventions the psychosocial wellbeing of those being treated actually improved

---

Reports on management from expert committees

- *Management of obesity in children and young people.* Guideline No 69 from SIGN (Scottish Intercollegiate Guidelines Network), 2003. www.sign.ac.uk/guidelines/fulltext/69/index.html (accessed 18 Oct)
- Summerbell CD, Waters E, Edmunds LD, Kelly S, Brown T, Campbell KJ. Interventions for preventing obesity in children. *Cochrane Database Syst Rev* 2005;(3):CD001871.
- Summerbell CD, Ashton V, Campbell KJ, Edmunds L, Kelly S, Waters E. Interventions for treating obesity in children. *Cochrane Database Syst Rev* 2005;(3):CD001872.
- Canadian review of reviews 2004. www.irsc.gc.ca/e/23293.html.
- *Clinical practice guidelines for the management of overweight and obesity in children and adolescents.* Australian review and evidence based guidelines. www.obesityguidelines.gov.au.
- Gibson P, Edmunds L, Haslam DW, Poskitt E. An approach to weight management in children and adolescents in primary care. *J Fam Health Care* 2002;12:108-9.
- Barlow SE, Dietz WH. Obesity evaluation and treatment: expert committee recommendations. *Pediatrics* 1998;102:E29.

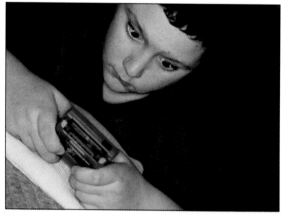

Time spent playing computer games may need to be reduced if an obese child is to achieve and maintain weight loss

---

Families can measure television viewing and related sedentary behaviours; if they reduce their viewing, this may result in them also reducing their food intake and increasing their physical activity

What should treatment aim for?

Weight maintenance over six to 12 months is considered to be a success, particularly as continued excessive weight gain is common in the absence of treatment. Weight maintenance is also successful because, with growth, paediatric patients can to some extent "grow into their weight."

Weight loss is an unrealistic aim except if patients have achieved prolonged weight maintenance or are severely obese and so have to lose weight to enable management of comorbidity such as type 2 diabetes or sleep apnoea. Progress with management should be reviewed with the family using the BMI centile chart periodically.

The photographs of adolescent girls and of a child playing a computer game are published with permission from Bubbles and Gusto/SPL respectively.

Aims of treatment

- To resolve comorbidity if it is present
- To achieve weight maintenance, not weight loss
- To ensure that families monitor their own diet, activity, television viewing, and computer use
- To introduce dietary changes
- To reduce sedentary behaviour (particularly television viewing)—to less than two hours a day
- To increase physical activity through lifestyle changes such as walking to and from school

Further reading

- Neovius M, Linne Y, Barkeling B, Rossner S. Discrepancies between classification systems of childhood obesity. *Obes Rev* 2004;52:105-14.
- Rudolf MCJ. The obese child. *Arch Dis Child Educ Pract* 2004;89:ep57-62. (http://adc.bmjjournals.com/).
- Viner R, Nicholls D. Managing obesity in secondary care. *Arch Dis Child* 2005;90:385-90.
- Stewart L, Houghton J, Hughes AR, Pearson D, Reilly JJ. Dietetic management of pediatric overweight: development and description of an evidence-based, behavioral, approach. *J Am Diet Assoc* 2005;105:1810-5.
- Kopelman PG, Caterson ID, Dietz WH, eds. *Clinical obesity in adults and children.* 2nd ed. Malden, MA: Blackwell, 2005.

12   Obesity—can we turn the tide?

Mike Lean, Laurence Gruer, George Alberti, Naveed Sattar

Recent headlines highlighting the current and projected obesity levels in the United Kingdom—in 2010 a third of adults will be obese—reiterate the cry that "it's time to do something about it." As already shown in this series, the consequences of obesity affect all ages and nearly all organ systems. Obesity diminishes quality of life, and many problems begin well before reaching a body mass index of 30. Well over half the entire population of the UK have a BMI of >25, and they will experience greater morbidity and total mortality.

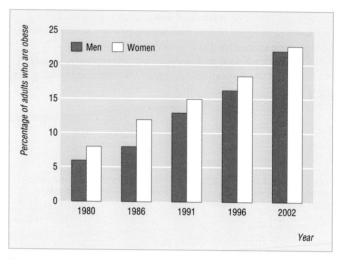

Trends in obesity in adults in England, 1980-2002 (graph adapted from *Health Survey for England 2004*). Projected levels suggest that by 2010 nearly a third of adult men and 28% of women in England will be obese (*Forecasting obesity to 2010*, www.dh.gov.uk/). The figures will be higher for older people

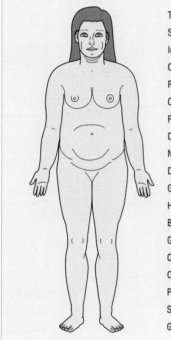

Medical complications of obesity

- Tiredness, depression
- Stroke
- Idiopathic intracranial hypertension
- Cataracts
- Pulmonary disease
- Coronary heart disease
- Pancreatitis
- Diabetes
- Non-alcoholic fatty liver disease
- Dyslipidaemia
- Gall bladder disease
- Hypertension
- Back pain
- Gynaecological abnormalities
- Cancers at many sites
- Osteoarthritis
- Phlebitis
- Skin disorders
- Gout

The problem of rising prevalence in obesity may get much worse—rates could climb still further, bankrupting the health system and leading soon to reductions in life expectancy. So, can we offer effective management? And can we reverse the rising trend in the prevalence of obesity, and if so, when?

Whose responsibility?

Although the old attitude of "pull yourself together, eat less, and exercise more" is receding, it is still evident among less perceptive health professionals and is commonly voiced by the media. Most overweight or obese individuals would prefer to be normal weight, and many are doing as much as they can to keep their weight lower than it would otherwise be.

We are all to some extent addicted to food. As with any disorder, people with excessive addiction to food require help, advice, and sympathy. Many become caught in a negative cycle of excess energy intake, continuing weight gain, and impaired appetite regulation, with physical inactivity an inevitable compounding factor.

People clearly have some responsibility for their health, but society and government have a responsibility to make the preferred, easy choices healthier ones. Health professionals have a responsibility to treat patients with understanding and sympathy and to call for changes in the food and activity environments to support improvements in public health.

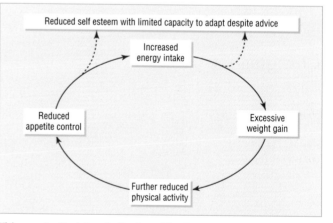

Vicious cycle of weight gain. Food provides short term pleasure and is addictive

It is increasingly apparent that most individuals are unable to make enough "proactive" changes to prevent excess weight gain but are simply "reactive" to their environment. Thus education alone will fail to halt this obesity epidemic, and environmental changes (physical, food, and fiscal policy) are urgently needed

Lessons from other countries

More attention could usefully be paid to the trends and differences in and between countries. Economic analyses show that recent increases in energy intake may be the predominant cause of increasing obesity, with physical inactivity playing an early facilitating but now compounding role. For example, in the United States, dependence on motorised transport, automated appliances in the home and workplace, and television viewing was established by 1970. However, obesity rates only began to accelerate in the '80s and '90s. This coincided with steady increases in food production and decreases in relative food costs, combined with more snacking and eating away from the home and consuming energy dense foods that are provided in ever bigger portions. The same trend now exists in other countries.

The real goal: prevention

Maintaining a stable weight is easier than losing excess weight. Indeed, a third to a half of all obese patients will not lose weight by any medical method. Much more effort should focus on discovering how to prevent individuals becoming overweight or obese in the first place and maintaining current weight. Prevention is the only economic long term solution to the problem. Even a complete understanding of the genes and peptide cascades that regulated appetite and metabolism can never reverse an epidemic driven by environmental and cultural change.

Relative contributions of diet and physical activity in achieving weight loss or weight maintenance

	Weight loss (big changes: ≥500 kcal/day)	Maintenance and prevention of weight gain (small changes: 50-100 kcal/day)
Diet alone	Substantial	Modest
Physical activity alone	Absent or minor	Modest
Diet and physical activity combined	Substantial	Substantial

Changing the obesogenic environment

If environments—physical, food, fiscal, and social environments—have become highly obesogenic, can they be changed? Although this has not yet happened anywhere, food consumption patterns can be adapted to enable people to satisfy both energy needs and taste buds without much conscious thought.

This can be facilitated by altering our physical activity environment. But changes are also needed both in the practices of the food industry and in the attitudes and behaviour of the public. Only small changes are needed, but it is difficult to imagine this all happening without an agency dedicated to combating obesity—with multifaceted specialist inputs and high level political influence.

Food industry and government

The 2002 joint consultation of the Food and Agriculture Organization of the United Nations and the World Health Organization used a systematic approach to published evidence to rank possible interventions. This ranking may, however, be misleading because comparable research efforts have not been

> **Rates of adult obesity in the Japanese and the French are strikingly lower than in the US and the UK, despite no evidence that they are more physically active. Their food cultures, however, are very different. Traditional ways of providing and eating food—such as families eating together at table—persist, albeit under threat from globalised catering, especially among young people**

What we can reasonably do about obesity now?*

- Establish a dedicated central agency responsible for all aspects of obesity nationally
- Develop a scoring system for obesogenicity of neighbourhoods, workplaces, and at or near schools
- Make certified training in obesity and weight management available for all healthcare professionals
- Fund evidenced based weight management in UK primary care
- Teach energy balance in all primary schools and disseminate information to all parents
- Encourage physical education for all school pupils, and use of school facilities out of school hours
- Ensure a health check (including body mass index and waist measurement) for all school leavers, both primary and secondary
- Display energy content of all meals and snacks at retail and catering outlets, with a warning if >700 kcals or >250 kcals, respectively
- Display saturated fat content of all ready meals and snacks at all retail and catering outlets, with a warning if >10% of total energy
- Allow new urban roads only if they have safe cycle lanes
- Allow new housing complexes only if they have sports facilities and green park areas
- Include helpline numbers for advice with all clothes sold with waist >102 cm for men; >94 cm for boys; >88 cm or size >16 for women; >80 cm for girls
- Ban advertising of slimming services without independent evaluation
- Ban television advertising of sweets and energy dense snacks and drinks before 9 pm and regulate all marketing to children
- Ban placement of sweets and energy dense snacks and drinks at or near shop tills and at child's eye level
- Fund adequate, effective obesity surgery in NHS for people with a body mass index of >40 facing disability
- Tax processed foods that are high in sugar or saturated fat, and reinvest that money in effective measures to increase intake of fruit, vegetables, and other low fat foods
- Introduce tax breaks for genuine corporate social responsibility to help avoid obesity by changes in food or activity environment
- Launch a health promotion campaign on the methods and benefits of weight maintenance and 5-10 kg weight loss

*The effectiveness of any adopted measures should be evaluated using continuous improvement methods

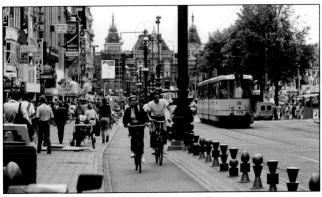

In the drive against rising obesity, new roads should be allowed only if they have safe cycle lanes, similar to those common in the Netherlands

43

applied to these or to other, potentially valuable measures. Furthermore, individual interventions may not be effective in isolation.

The food industry is the largest, most powerful industry of all; food is essential for life and health, and the industry must remain profitable. The industry is largely driven by commercial forces aimed at maximising consumption and hence profit. Given people's increasing reliance on processed and precooked food, the industry needs to assume much more responsibility for preventing obesity. Governments, as custodians of public health, have keys roles in creating the conditions for this to happen. Voluntary agreements have not been enough. Foods that are less energy dense are needed; this would reduce the total energy content of what is sold and eaten in meals and snacks, without reintroducing calories in other foods.

What is provided determines what is eaten, and so what is provided has to change. This will require attention to pricing and marketing policies, product design, portion sizes, energy content and density, and customer information. Moreover, the advertising of energy dense foods needs to be substantially curtailed—"out of sight, out of mind" holds especially true for children.

The Treaty of Rome included the principle that public health consequences should be considered for all decisions made in public life: ministers can no longer ignore this issue. We need effective regulations or active support and incentives for measures that reflect "corporate social responsibility."

Education

For the public
The measures outlined above may not succeed unless the public is also persuaded to change its dietary and physical behaviour. Intensive efforts, supported by government, are also needed to change the prevailing food and drink culture.

A reasonable educational target for the near future might be to teach the simplest principles of energy balance at primary school level. But education alone may have only a limited effect, and even that is likely to be mainly among those best able to assimilate knowledge. The highest obesity levels seem to be among those in the most deprived socioeconomic areas, particularly in women (although many factors other than knowledge are relevant here). Education is essential at all levels—for children and adults, and for policy planners.

More innovative ways of educating the public, including children, are clearly needed. The media also have a role in disseminating messages and must be trained appropriately.

For health professionals
Historically, nutrition has been poorly taught to doctors, but the General Medical Council's *Tomorrow's Doctors* initiative has urged improvements in nutrition education for medical undergraduates.

A strong case now exists for making obesity a core part of all medical curriculums and part of the training of all other health professions. Continuing emphasis should be placed on obesity in postgraduate teaching—both in the early generic professional training programmes for all specialties and then later in relevant specialty programmes. In other words, any contact between a medical professional and a patient is an opportunity to assess whether that patient has a weight problem—and to offer advice.

Embracing obesity treatments

Some issues peculiar to obesity remain complex—for example, what constitutes success for medical interventions against

Summary of strength of evidence on factors that might promote or protect against weight gain and obesity. Source: Food and Agriculture Organization of the United Nations

Strength of evidence	Factors protecting against obesity	Factors promoting obesity
Convincing	Regular physical activity; high intake of dietary fibre	Sedentary lifestyles; high intake of foods high in energy and poor in micronutrients
Probable	Home and school environments that support healthy food choices for children; breast feeding	Heavy marketing of energy dense foods and fastfood outlets; high intake of sugars (sweetened soft drinks and fruit juices); adverse socioeconomic conditions (in developed countries, especially for women)
Possible*	Foods with low glycaemic index	Large portion sizes; high proportion of food prepared outside home (developed countries); eating patterns showing "rigid restraint and periodic disinhibition"
Insufficient	Increased frequency of eating	Alcohol

*Possible evidence also exists that the protein content of a diet has no effect on weight gain and obesity.

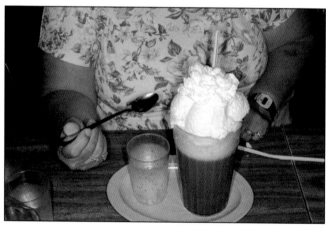

Can people be persuaded to eat smaller portions, abandon energy dense soft drinks, and drink less alcohol? Can they be persuaded to walk more?

Obesity affects all branches of medicine and surgery, and all doctors can contribute to its treatment and prevention either directly or by appropriate referral

Training courses in obesity
- In the UK, the postgraduate intercollegiate course on nutrition offers an introduction to obesity for doctors
- Internationally, the International Obesity Task Force (part of the International Association for the Study of Obesity) has introduced postgraduate training in the SCOPE (Specialist Certification of Obesity Professional in Europe) programme

obesity. The goals of public health planners (such as halving the rate of weight gain and reducing the prevalence of obesity related diseases) do not easily translate into management targets for individuals' weight loss and maintenance. Even the internationally accepted target for weight loss (5-10 kg)—which confers a high proportion of the potential medical benefit, through loss of intra-abdominal fat—is rarely acceptable to patients.

The UK now has safe, effective adjunctive drug treatments that are approved by the National Institute for Health and Clinical Excellence, and evidence based surgical methods for obesity are also available. Routine health care now offers evidenced based, structured multidisciplinary management of obesity. In the UK, Counterweight (an obesity management project in selected general practices around the country) is a good example.

Not all patients are willing or able to participate fully in such programmes, but for over half of those who do, quite modest, achievable weight loss brings major benefits for obesity related diseases in every system of the body. Once a weight management programme is established, we have a duty to evaluate and improve the programme. Doctors, patients, and healthcare providers must recognise the costs of not providing effective weight management.

New research

Health services and governments need to realise that the research conducted so far has not answered all the essential questions. Researchers have tended to focus on the efficacy and safety of interventions. Much more research is needed on routine services in community and population settings to provide a basis for future interventions. There is also a need for continuous evaluation of current policies, commercial practices, and cultural attitudes to help in the understanding of current trends in and between countries and to shape improved approaches. New research skills, new methods, and new funding pathways are needed.

Conclusions

Medical practice must adapt to the current epidemic of obesity and nutrition related diseases. The profession must unite the forces of public health and acute services to generate sustainable changes in food and lifestyles, matters at the heart of our cultural identities. Furthermore, training in public health medicine should urge all doctors to contribute towards bringing changes in the food industry and in the environment that will lead to a more physically active, healthier, and happier population.

Society has accepted long term expensive drug treatments to reduce risks from preventable conditions such as type 2 diabetes, hypertension, and coronary heart disease. To be consistent, it must accept that many people now need drugs (and in some cases, surgery) to cut risks of and disability from obesity, and to limit its progression.

As the prevalence and costs of obesity escalate, the economic argument for giving high priority to obesity and weight management through a designated coordinating agency will ultimately become overwhelming. The only question is, will action be taken before it's too late?

The photographs of cycle lanes, ice cream drink, and swimming are published with permission from Martin Bond/Alamy, Martin Parr/Magnum, and SIPA/Rex respectively.

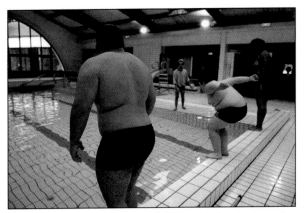
Swimming is good for flexibility, but daily "weight bearing leg use" (walking, running, and even standing) is more valuable

In the Counterweight programme, patients have six appointments or group sessions over three months, with follow-up sessions every three months for one year then annual reviews. The aim is to achieve at least 5-10 kg weight loss, then weight maintenance—the success rate in the programme so far is about 30-40%. The programme is continuously evaluated and improved

Future research into obesity and its prevention
- Research questions from observational studies
- Basic science research on mechanisms in the inter-regulation of eating and physical activity, and subsequent clinical trials (phase I translational research)
- Controlled family and community interventions and evaluation of population directed policy measures (phase II translational research)
- Research on generating supportive environmental changes (physical, food, fiscal, and educational environments) and continuous improvement evaluation (phase III translational research, for sustainability)

*Adapted from Hiss (ww.niddk.nih.gov/fund/other/Diabetes-Translation/conf-publication.pdf) and Petticrew and Roberts (*J Epidemiol Comm Health* 2003;57:527-9)

Further reading and resources
- World Health Organization and Food and Agricultural Organisation of the United Nations. *Diet, nutrition and the prevention of chronic diseases.* 2002. www.fao.org/docrep/005/AC911E/AC911E00.htm
- International obesity taskforce (www.iotf.org/)
- Counterweight—a multicentre obesity management project led by practice nurses, conducted in 80 general practices in seven regions of the UK (www.counterweight.org)
- SCOPE programme (www.iotf.org/media/scoperelease.htm)
- Intercollegiate Course on Human Nutrition (www.icgnutrition.org.uk/coursedet.rtf)
- International Association for the Study of Obesity. Guiding principles for reducing the commercial promotion of foods and beverages to children ("Sydney principles"). www.iotf.org/sydneyprinciples/index.asp

Index